Thrive Through Yoga

For the day dreamers, trail blazers and magic trusters.
For the black sheep and odd ducks and those with messy hair and even messier hearts.
For those who loved me in my darkest moments and helped me navigate my way out of the depths.
And for you Dad. For inspiring me to be fearless and share my soul with the world.
I'll see you on the other side of the stars.

Thrive Through Yoga

A 21-Day Journey to Ease Anxiety, Love Your Body and Feel More Alive

Nicola Jane Hobbs

B L O O M S B U R Y

LONDON · OXFORD · NEW YORK · NEW DELHI · SYDNEY

Green Tree
An imprint of Bloomsbury Publishing Plc

50 Bedford Square
London
WC1B 3DP
UK

1385 Broadway
New York
NY 10018
USA

www.bloomsbury.com

BLOOMSBURY and the Diana logo are trademarks of Bloomsbury Publishing Plc

First published in 2018
© Nicola Jane Hobbs, 2018

British Library Cataloguing-in-Publication Data
A catalogue record for this book is available from the British Library.

ISBN: Paperback: 9781472942999
ePub: 9781472943019
ePDF: 9781472943002

2 4 6 8 10 9 7 5 3 1

Typeset in Myriad and Klinic Slab by Louise Millar
Printed and bound in China by C&C Offset Printing Co.

All photography by Glen Burrows Photography,
with the exception of images on pages 88, 100 © Getty Images
Illustrations by Matt Windsor

Bloomsbury Publishing Plc makes every effort to ensure that the papers used in the manufacture
of our books are natural, recyclable products made from wood grown in well-managed forests.
Our manufacturing processes conform to the environmental regulations of the country of origin.

To find out more about our authors and books visit www.bloomsbury.com. Here you will find extracts,
author interviews, details of forthcoming events and the option to sign up for our newsletters.

Contents

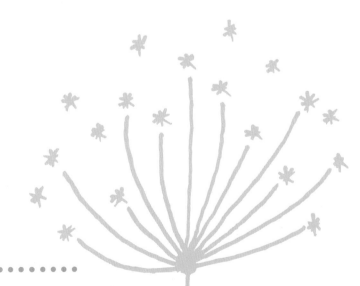

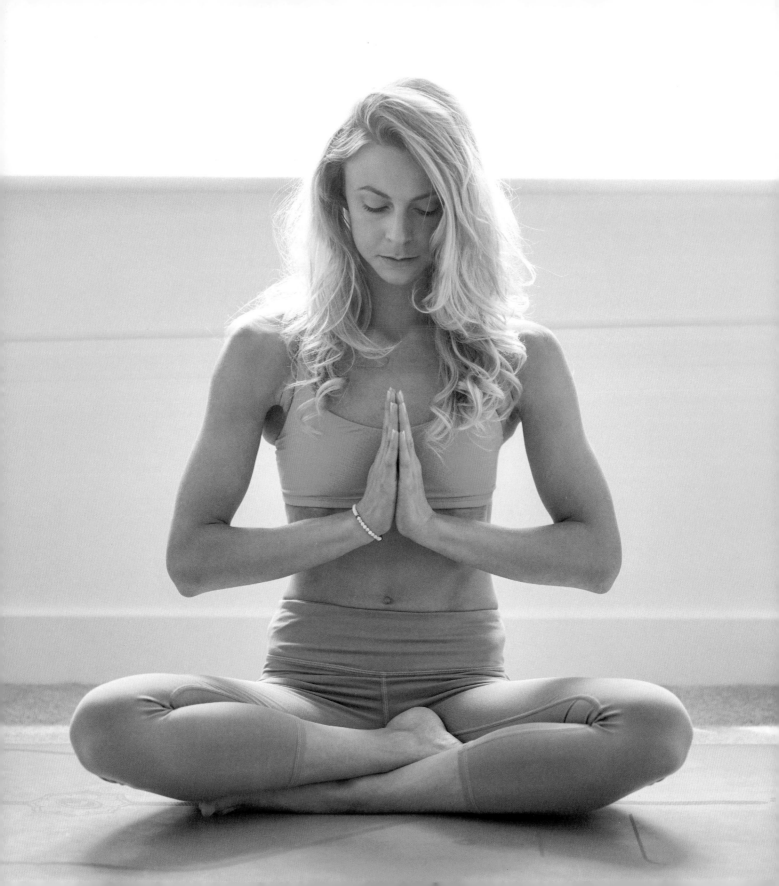

Part 1: Introduction

The purpose of yoga is not to put your foot behind your head. Or do the splits. Or perfect a handstand. Yoga is about more than pretty poses. It's about healing. Thriving. Understanding what it means to be truly alive. The purpose of yoga is to find freedom where you were once trapped. To open your heart to joy and adventure. To make peace with your body. To accept yourself completely. To become aware of all the beautiful things about you. And to restore your soul with kindness and compassion so you can serve others from the overflow. The true purpose of yoga is love. To love your body, yourself and the world.

This book was created from that love. My aim is to take you on a journey of transformation. To give you a blueprint to thrive. Because I want to create change. To create hope. I want you to begin this quest as you are – you don't need to be more together or more falling apart. Just come exactly as you are. And, over the next 21 days, I will take you on a journey designed to help you grow as bold and as a brave and as beautiful as you were born to be.

The *Thrive Through Yoga* journey has been created from my personal experiences, professional practice, ancient wisdom, and modern science. It will begin by introducing you to what thriving is and how it can help us heal from some of the common struggles we face in 21st-century life. It will move on to outline some of the key concepts of yoga, and answer frequently asked questions to help you understand why I have chosen to include different elements of yoga, psychology and spirituality in the journey. You will then be introduced to the Thrive Sequence – a routine you will practise most days as a form of moving meditation.

Then we'll begin our 21-day journey where each day you will find a quote to inspire you, yoga routine, heart-centred exploration and meditation. You will also find yoga sequences for common struggles such as insomnia, stress and anxiety towards the back of the book, along with a Yoga Pose Library which will give you instructions on how to practise each pose safely.

But first I would like to start with my promise to you – from writer to reader, teacher to student, soul to soul…

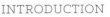

My promises to you

- I promise that you are capable and worthy of thriving.

- I promise that you have suffered long enough. You don't have to haul your struggles around any longer. Whatever is controlling you or holding you back, it's time to let it go.

- I promise that you will always make it through. You will heal one day. It will happen when you least expect it and you won't even notice it when it does. One day you will wake up and realise that you aren't pretending any more. You aren't fighting or striving or hustling for worthiness. You will realise you are free.

- I promise that you can unlearn all the stuff that makes you stressed and angry and scared. When you take off your mask and reveal yourself you will begin to find freedom. You will un-become everything that isn't really you, so you can become everything that you are meant to be.

- I promise that your fear, your loneliness and all your struggles are fragile. A song, a poem, a sunset, a hug can cause you to break open and it will obliterate them into insignificance. At any moment your struggles can shatter into nothingness. They have no more power than that.

- I promise that you feel pain so that the smallest joys in your life appear bigger. You experience loss so that you can appreciate the people that touch your heart. It rains so that you can delight in the beauty of the sun. You're not supposed to be happy all the time. Life hurts. Life is hard. Your pain has a purpose.

- I promise that by facing the fear and uncertainty in your life you will free yourself from it. When you don't allow yourself to embrace your hurt, and instead numb it or dismiss it or medicate it, you miss the lessons in your suffering. It is these lessons that will heal your soul and help you grow.

- I promise that you will reach a point where you will wake up to the beauty of life. You will look back at who you used to be and it will hurt because you will realise that you neglected yourself for so long. You will heal. You will grow. You will evolve. You will become more loving and more compassionate. And you will help the world become a better place.

- I promise that making peace with your past, doing what makes your soul happy and living with an open heart will transform your life. It won't be easy, but it will be the most important thing you ever do. When you open your heart to love, magic and unimaginable adventures you will begin to discover that life is beautiful.

- I promise that love is more important than fear.

- I promise that it is your time to thrive.

My story

I have written this book because it is the book I needed when I was younger. At a time when I felt lost and scared and totally alone.

I know what it feels like to live with a broken soul. To feel worthless and empty, and too damaged to love. To feel like you have no voice, that the world is too loud, and that there is no way out of this cycle of struggle and self-hate.

But there is a way out. Because I also know what it is like to feel freedom. To feel worthy and loved and full of life. To feel strong and healthy and proud of who you are. I know what it feels like to be grateful for your body and to enjoy nourishing it. To feel like you are someone of value. To be happy. To climb mountains, do cartwheels, and experience life becoming more magical each day.

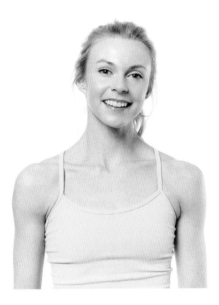

As a child I always felt a little different, like I didn't quite belong. I had a happy life on the outside – a loving family, great friends, good grades … but I felt disconnected, misunderstood and lost. I didn't know how to communicate this vulnerability, this anxiety, this hurt, so I started starving myself. Because hunger felt better than hurt.

I was diagnosed with anorexia nervosa, depression, anxiety and obsessive compulsive disorder when I was 15. These labels kept me trapped in a cycle of psychiatric admissions and hospital refeeding regimes for the next five years. I was given therapy, put on drugs and force fed. But each time I was discharged from hospital I was left feeling disempowered, worthless and hating food, my body and myself even more.

At 19, weighing 25kg, I ended up with organ failure. Depressed, drained and defeated, I had two choices. To give up. Or to do something remarkable with my life.

I chose life.

Over the next two years, I regained weight, health and strength. I then went on to finish my psychology degree, travel to Thailand to train as a yoga teacher, complete a Master's degree in sport and exercise psychology, become two times English Champion in Olympic weightlifting, build a yoga business, write my first book, *Yoga Gym*, and train in Ayurvedic nutrition and lifestyle consultancy.

After you almost kill yourself, you can't go back to being the way you were. I used to dream of being a top lawyer or having some high-flying corporate career with a posh house, big paycheck and designer handbag, but my near-death experience shook me awake. It showed me my limitations, addictions and all the things that were holding me back. It demolished my ego and broke my heart wide open. I became so desperate that I had no other choice but to transform my life.

I feel a responsibility to not let my pain have been in vain. So now my focus is on helping people to thrive – through yoga, writing, psychology and Ayurveda. These are the practices that helped me to heal, find freedom and feel love.

And I want you to feel that love too.

Nicola x

The aim of *Thrive Through Yoga*

Thrive Through Yoga is a revolutionary route to freedom that can help liberate you from the anxieties and worries of modern life and help you transform into a happy, confident and resilient person.

It doesn't matter how long you've been struggling with stress, anxiety or low self-esteem, or what disorders you've been labelled with: when you've got the support, inspiration and dream for freedom, you can start living in a way that will help you become the person you yearn to become – the wild, passionate, sparkly-eyed person with love in your heart and adventure in your spirit that you've been hiding for so long.

For years I was told I would never recover. I was told I would always have depression and need to be on medication, and that the eating disorder would always be with me and I would just have to manage it. But I believe that everyone is capable of finding freedom and happiness, of liberating themselves from anxiety, fear and anger, and of feeling love and compassion for themselves and the world.

So, my mission is to help you emerge from the storms of your broken soul twice as strong, graceful and independent as before. Whether you're struggling with anxiety or stress, going through an eating disorder or depression, or just feeling generally fed up with life, I want to give you the tools to heal and to thrive.

Thrive Through Yoga has three main aims:

- **To help you develop a daily practice of self-care.** It is not selfish to take care of yourself and make your happiness a priority. *Thrive Through Yoga* will teach you the importance of caring for yourself. Just as you clean your teeth every morning, nourishing yourself through yoga, meditation and relaxation will become part of your daily routine. By making the time to look after your own wellbeing, you will have the energy and love to share with others.

- **To help you let go of anything that no longer nourishes you.** Often when we are going through stress, anxiety or struggle we are malnourished – physically, mentally, emotionally and spiritually. *Thrive Through Yoga* uses a variety of yoga sequences, meditations and heart-centred explorations to build physical strength and nourish you emotionally.

- **To help strengthen the bodymind.** In the Eastern world the body and mind are seen as a single "bodymind". We cannot influence the body without simultaneously affecting what we think and how we feel. *Thrive Through Yoga* uses yoga sequences to build strength and flexibility, which will also create psychological resilience and emotional freedom.

What is the bodymind?

In the West we commonly treat the mind and body as separate, while the bodymind approach views them as a single unit. The brain is an anatomical structure found in the head, whereas the mind is a stream of consciousness found throughout the whole body. It includes our ability to think, perceive, reason and feel, and flows through every cell in our body. This is an Eastern approach traditionally found in Buddhism, but modern medicine is starting to recognise the unity of body and mind through psychoneuroimmunology (the study of the interaction between psychological processes, emotions, and the nervous and immune systems), and psychosomatic medicine (a medical field exploring the relationship between mental, social, behavioural and bodily processes).

Research has found that emotional energy causes neuropeptides to be released from cells that cause physiological reactions in our body. This is why the *Thrive Through Yoga* journey involves emotional release via yoga poses – to literally release issues trapped in the tissues.

What is thriving?

The teenager who lost his leg in a car accident and went on to win Gold in the Paralympics is thriving. The mother who at first felt despair when she found out her son had autism, then trained as a coach to help other parents going through a similar situation is thriving. The man who was on the verge of suicide after being made redundant and went on to launch a service to help those without a job rebuild their self-worth is thriving. The woman who feels constantly anxious, exhausted and not good enough, who transforms herself so she can be more compassionate towards herself and the world is thriving.

We all go through challenges in life. It may be a divorce, a death of a loved one, a physical or mental illness or a stressful job. When we face challenges like these, one of two things usually happens:

- We remain devastated by them.

- We grow stronger from them – we thrive.

I first discovered the concept of thriving when I was writing the thesis for my Master's degree in sport and exercise psychology. I studied the subject partly because yoga had been one of the things that helped me to heal and I wanted to understand what it was about yoga that was so transformational.

The more research I did, the more I discovered stories of people who had not only overcome struggles in their lives, but had actually grown stronger from them. These people had transformed their struggles into strength. The pain, fear and adversity which could have caused them to crumble, instead awakened new strength and wisdom within them and inspired them to blossom.

Over the past few years, thriving has become particularly interesting to researchers. Whereas depression, illness and despair used to dominate research, happiness, hope and personal growth is beginning to take precedence.

In 1996, two psychologists, Professor Lawrence Calhoun and Dr. Richard Tedeschi, based at the University of North Carolina, developed the Post Traumatic Growth Inventory – a measure that assesses how people have grown stronger from their struggles. They found five elements that reflect thriving:

- Discovery of new paths and possibilities.

- New ways of relating to others.

- Increases in personal strength.

- Spiritual change.

- A greater appreciation of life.

Often, it is not until we are struggling with some aspect of our life that we begin to look deeply at ourselves and realise what truly matters.

So, this is my definition of thriving:

Thrive
(v.) To transform struggle into strength; to grow in knowledge, confidence and compassion; to feel hope, connection and belonging; to live and love with your whole heart; to blossom; to flourish; to become alive.

From this definition, combined with previous research and my own experience, I have created the **T.H.R.I.V.E.** model: six steps we can go through in order to move from struggle to strength.

Take responsibility – the more responsibility we are able to take for our life, the more we are going to be able to create the future that we want.

Have hope – hope never abandons us but sometimes, in times of struggle, we find ourselves abandoning it. At this stage we find hope within ourselves. Even at the darkest of moments we can choose to feel hope.

Recreate yourself – our struggles often become part of our identity. In order to find freedom, we need to let go of our previous sense of self and establish who we truly want to be.

Initiate action – you can't think your way to freedom. When we are going through struggle, we often spend years formulating a plan without making any real changes in our lives. At this stage we will begin changing the way we act on a daily basis in order to diminish fear, anxiety and insecurity.

Value change – change is scary, but if our lives were exactly the same in 10 years' time then we would probably be disappointed and unhappy. At this stage we learn how to value change as a reflection of our personal growth.

Enjoy the journey – not everything worthwhile has to involve pain and suffering. At this stage we find ways to allow ourselves to enjoy our journey. Although thriving takes time and effort, it doesn't mean we can't have as much fun as possible along the way.

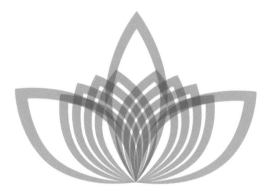

What is the difference between thriving and self-improvement?
Thrive Through Yoga is not just some kind of self-improvement project or ideal we're trying to live up to. When we begin a journey of transformation we often focus on self-improvement and convince ourselves that we would be a better person if we could eat healthier, meditate more or drop a dress size. But thriving does not entail this conditional self-acceptance or subtle self-aggression. Thriving involves accepting who we are which creates space for us to grow. It's not about throwing ourselves away to become better. It's about making friends with who we are. We can still feel scared or angry or not good enough and learn to love who we are and all our imperfections and unwanted parts. And it is with this loving kindness that we will begin to grow.

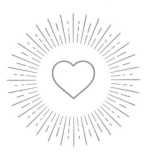

Disorders, disease and distress

The opposite of thriving is suffering. It is stress, struggle, disorder and disease. If you are reading this book it is likely there is something in your life that you are struggling with. It may be a mental illness like depression or anorexia, a build-up of stress and anxiety from work, or a vague feeling of discomfort that things aren't quite right.

Below is a list of ten of the most common struggles that many of us face in 21st-century life. It is helpful to understand signs of disorder and distress in ourselves and others, so we can seek professional help if we need to.

I asked people who were going through these struggles what they actually felt like, so if you can relate to some of the feelings and experiences described this is nothing to be ashamed of. Just remember, these struggles are engines for transformation. They are the springboards that will launch you on your journey to find new meaning, purpose, and direction in your life.

If you do feel like you are struggling with any of the issues below, please seek professional help. You are not alone.

Depression

Depression is one of the most common mental health disorders worldwide. While it is normal to feel depressed at difficult times in our lives such as losing a loved one, going through a divorce, or getting fired from a job, sometimes the sadness and loneliness persists and makes it difficult to carry on with daily functioning.

Having been through depression myself, I would say it feels like a big black cloud that masks the beauty of the sun. It feels like your wings have been clipped so you can no longer fly. It feels like you have a 10-tonne ball of lead in your chest that you've got no choice but to drag around with you. It feels like you have lost yourself.

Depression may come and go or you may feel like it all the time. It may be a mild sadness or you may feel it really powerfully. No matter how intensely you feel the depression, it's important to talk to someone and get help so you can fly freely again.

Anxiety

Like depression, anxiety is one of the most common mental health issues globally with over eight million people experiencing an anxiety disorder in the UK each year.

Anxiety feels like your mind is on fire, like your thoughts are running wild and bumping into each other. It feels like there is a phone buzzing in your head that never stops ringing. It feels like a constant tidal wave of thoughts, worries, and emotions that make your heart flutter, your stomach knot and your breath quicken.

People experience anxiety about different things and in different ways. Some people are anxious about social situations or have certain phobias, while others have panic attacks or more general anxiety and worries.

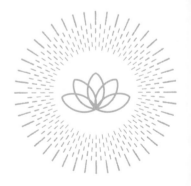

Stress

Modern life is full of demands and deadlines and, for many of us, feeling stressed has become a way of life. Over half of us admit to feeling stressed on a daily basis. While stress can be a great motivator and help us perform well under pressure, it can become overwhelming and begin to affect our health, relationships and quality of life.

Stress feels like we are under too much mental or emotional pressure. It feels like we are unable to bridge the gap between what people expect of us and what we can actually do. It feels like we are carrying the weight of the world on our shoulders, like we are being pulled in every direction, and like we are falling into an abyss and constantly looking for a rope to help us climb out.

Our body can't detect the difference between a life-threatening source of stress such as being chased by a bear, or a modern-life cause like a demanding work schedule, rocky relationship or money issues. And because modern causes of stress tend to be chronic, it means our body is in a constant state of fight-or-flight, even if there are no bears to run away from. The result is imbalance which can lead to heart disease, obesity, diabetes, headaches, insomnia and mental health problems.

Eating disorders and disordered eating

In 21st-century society there is a huge amount of focus on the way we look, and this affects our relationship with food and our body. Research has found that over six per cent of people in the UK have an eating disorder, increasing to 20 per cent of women between the ages of 16–24. Statistics also show that 55 per cent of us go on some sort of restrictive diet every year. Disordered eating is far more common than you think, and includes diagnosable disorders like anorexia, bulimia and binge eating disorder, as well as any form of overly restrictive eating, fasting, yo-yo dieting, obsessive calorie counting, so-called 'clean' eating and meal skipping that has a harmful effect on your mental, emotional or physical wellbeing.

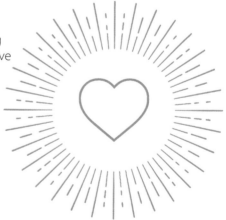

Speaking from personal experience, anorexia feels like you're in an abusive relationship with yourself. You feel like you can't control anything, so you control food because the real things in life are too difficult to deal with. So, you allow food and calories to occupy your mind instead. You feel you are not worthy of nourishment, so you punish yourself instead. You fool yourself that you are strong and that emptiness is power, when actually you feel weaker than you could ever imagine. Eating disorders are like a cosy little hell – familiar and secure but full of loneliness, fear and hurt.

For some people disordered eating can be a lifelong battle, so it's important to get out of your cosy little hell and seek professional support as soon as you realise your wellbeing and your life is being restricted by food.

Obsessive Compulsive Disorder (OCD)

Although OCD is considered the fourth most common mental illness, many people still suffer in silence because of shame. We can all be a little obsessive about things at times – maybe we like our desk arranged a certain way, or our house has to be spotless, or we have to check the front door is locked a couple of times before we leave for work. OCD is when these obsessions take over our life.

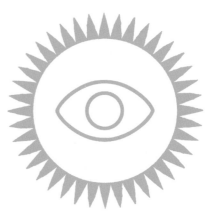

OCD feels like you need to flick the light switch 10 times or your family will die. It feels like you have to wash your hands 50 times or you are going to get ill, you have to eat exactly 127 cornflakes or something bad will happen, or you have to count your steps around the house so you'll be safe. It feels like you are going crazy because you are totally aware that your thoughts and rituals are irrational, but it is the only way you feel you can survive.

Like eating disorders, OCD becomes a cosy little hell. Even though freedom from OCD is possible, it is often treated as a lifelong condition because the unknown of resisting obsessions and compulsions often seems scarier than the familiarity of the disorder.

Addiction

Addiction is when you become enslaved to a habit. You can be addicted to a substance such as alcohol, or a behaviour such as gambling. There are well-known addictions like drugs and smoking, and then there are other addictions which are probably more common but less thought of as addictions – coffee, healthy food, junk food, shopping, social media, plastic surgery and exercise. We can even be addicted to work.

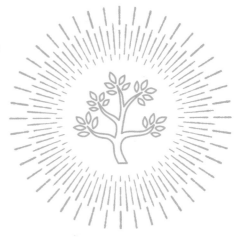

Addiction can mean that you're not awake until you've had your third cup of coffee, or you miss your mum's birthday meal because you were in the gym. It's lying about how many drinks you've had or sneaking a cigarette before a date. It's having to take a nap in the car on your lunchbreak because you stayed up until 3am on social media. It's starting the diet on Monday again and promising that you'll quit smoking 'some day'.

The substance or behaviour we are addicted to doesn't have to be dangerous in itself to become an addiction. However, when you give that substance or behaviour top priority in your life, or it makes you feel more in control, you find yourself becoming anxious or uncomfortable if you can't use it or do it, or it starts to disrupt your life and your relationships then it is time to ask for help.

Exhaustion

Despite statistics showing six out of seven of us wake up feeling exhausted, many of us feel ashamed to admit it in case other people think we can't cope.

We live in a 24/7 society where life seems to happen at breakneck speed and in order to keep up we compromise on sleep and relaxation. I remember a time when I was studying for my Master's degree, doing freelance journalism, setting up my first yoga business, commuting over 100 miles a day, and competing in Olympic weightlifting, all on four to five hours of sleep a night. A few months later I crashed with adrenal fatigue. I hear stories like mine all the time from people trying to juggle too much – kids, work, going to the gym, looking after parents, washing, cleaning… Sooner or later they crash.

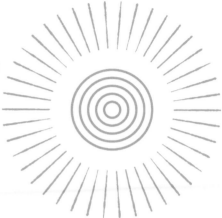

The exhaustion can be physical, mental, or emotional (or a combination of all three) and, without help, can eventually lead to a suppressed immune system and disorders such as Chronic Fatigue Syndrome (CFS).

Body shame

You only have to glance at social media to be inundated with images of what society deems as beautiful. These unattainable beauty ideals contribute to us feeling shame about our bodies. This is one of the biggest struggles of modern life with 90 per cent of us saying our body causes us to feel down and taints our enjoyment of everyday life.

On average we have 13 negative thoughts about our body a day. We tell ourselves that our thighs are fat, we hate our bellies, and that we have a big nose and bags under our eyes. We call ourselves 'fat' and 'ugly' and emotionally abuse ourselves on a daily basis.

But, even though we are targeting the size of our thighs or the wobble of our belly, our body is usually not to blame at all. I spent years hating my body and I learnt that whenever I was beating myself up over my stretchmarks or the flatness of my chest, it was because I'd had a bad day at work, an argument with my boyfriend, or I was feeling sad, scared, or confused about something else in my life.

I promise you that all the sit-ups in the world won't make you feel better about your stomach, because your stomach was never the problem to begin with.

Perfectionism and not enough-ness

We live in a culture of perfectionism, with 80 per cent of us feeling like we're not good enough – not thin enough, not pretty enough, not clever enough, not good enough partners, not good enough parents, not good enough at our jobs . . . Just not enough. Scientists have even given it a name: Atelophobia – the fear of imperfection and not being enough. This is a sign of low self-esteem and is closely related to other disorders such as depression, anxiety, self-harm and eating disorders.

For me, this feeling of not enough-ness fuelled my anorexia. I spent years disliking myself and feeling worthless. I would beat myself up for getting an A grade when an A* was possible. I aimed to be the perfect daughter, the perfect sister, the perfect student, all the time feeling like a failure. I even doubted I was thin enough to have anorexia at the same time as doubting whether I was really deserving of recovery and happiness. Only when I made peace with perfectionism, realised my worth, and learnt that I was unconditionally enough, did I find the courage to let go of the anorexia and start creating a life I loved.

Busy-o-holic

We all know what it's like to have a jam-packed calendar full of work, hobbies, chores, family gatherings and social events. At first it's exciting and the buzz of busy-ness gives us a rush. However, after a while, even though we might be craving some free time to relax, having white space on our calendar induces anxiety. And, if we do take some time out from our hectic lives, we feel guilty for not being productive.

We live in a culture that celebrates being busy and many of us feel like the more we do, the happier we will be. Society has conditioned us to believe that being busy equates to being successful. However, this urge to fill our free time with 'stuff' can be detrimental. It's often an escape or a way to numb ourselves.

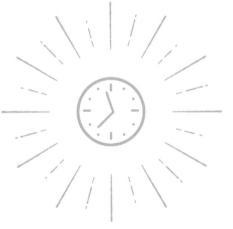

This compulsive busy-ness can be seen as an addiction or an obsession, or even a coping mechanism to deal with not feeling good enough. It's easy to see how it can lead to stress, anxiety, depression and other mental health issues.

This highlights how all these modern-day struggles are interlinked. If we can escape the cycle of just one of these struggles, it's likely we'll find freedom from others too.

How does *Thrive Through Yoga* work?

On my journey to freedom I explored a huge variety of therapies and treatments, ranging from cognitive behavioural therapy (CBT) and psychoanalysis, to reiki and spiritual healing. *Thrive Through Yoga* combines what I found most helpful on my personal journey as well as what I have found to be most effective through my yoga teaching and exercise psychology work, with evidence-based techniques to ease anxiety, improve self-worth and increase body confidence. You'll find a list of references at the back of the book with details of research studies and websites where you can find more information on certain topics.

In order to turn all this experience and research into something that you can incorporate into your daily life, *Thrive Through Yoga* simplifies the healing powers of yoga and ancient wisdom along with modern science and evidence-based psychological principles into a life-changing 21-day journey. It is a step-by-step guide that will give you the practical tools you need so that you can let go of whatever is holding you back – so you can thrive.

From stress-proofing your life and facing your fears, to easing anxiety and loving your body, each day will introduce you to a stepping stone on your journey to happiness and freedom. It will give you an inspirational quote, heart-centred exploration, meditation or aspiration, and yoga routine specific to the theme for that day. There is also a Thrive Sequence to repeat daily, to help you tune into your body and your breath, switch off from any stress or anxiety, and bring your awareness to the present moment.

For plants, the motivation towards growth is inbuilt. The same is true for humans. Imagine you are a plant and *Thrive Through Yoga* is your water and sunlight. It will give you daily nourishment so you can blossom and grow. The holistic approach of *Thrive Through Yoga* is based on the four methods and practices that follow.

How do inspirational quotes and mantras work?

Each day of the *Thrive Through Yoga* journey begins with an inspirational quote or mantra. The beautiful thing about inspirational quotes is that they show us that our struggles are shared. When we read a phrase or mantra that resonates with us we realise that we are not alone, that other people have been through what we are going through and have found the strength to keep going. Thriving is not just about knowledge but also about connection, and these quotes are powerful in helping us see something in ourselves that we want to overcome and giving us the hope and faith that change is possible.

What are heart-centred explorations?

Much of our learning and personal growth focuses on developing the mind instead of the heart. Heart-centred explorations use the power of the heart to transform our lives. They are similar to mindset exercises, only they move our awareness from our ego to our higher self and encourage us to move from living from a place of fear and comparison to love and compassion. By tuning into our hearts with these explorations we can start seeing beyond self-limiting beliefs related to our body, job, money and material possessions, and begin reconnecting with our true selves, rediscovering our passions and accepting and loving ourselves deeply and completely.

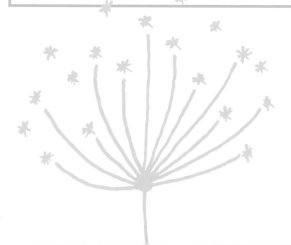

What is the difference between affirmations and aspirations?

Aspirations are used on many days of the *Thrive Through Yoga* journey. There is a subtle but profound difference between affirmations and aspirations. Affirmations are positive statements or declarations that will something into being, e.g. 'I love my body'. Aspirations are a willingness to be open to a new way of being e.g. 'May I love my body'. Affirmations are popular in self-help and personal development books, however research shows that they can backfire because we find that the statements we are telling ourselves are so unbelievable that it creates conflict in our mind, and our negative beliefs become stronger. For example, if deep down we see ourselves as ugly but we affirm, 'I am beautiful and I love myself', we create an inner war because we don't genuinely believe in what we are saying. If, however, we use an aspiration such as, 'May I see myself as beautiful and learn to love myself', instead of forcing change upon us which leads to resistance, we invite change with softness and openness allowing us to be more loving towards ourselves so natural growth can take place.

1 – Yoga

Like me, a lot of people come to yoga because they have a storm brewing inside them. Maybe they are stressed or anxious, or they are numbing out their feelings with food, TV or work, or they just want to feel more alive. Others come because they want to reconnect with a part of themselves they feel they have lost touch with, or to connect with something deeper they don't fully understand.

Most therapies focus on the mind, but I feel that one of the first steps to healing is through the body. From my own journey, I can say that reconnecting with my body through yoga was one of the most powerful practices that ignited recovery from my struggles. Using a variety of strengthening yang poses and relaxing yin poses, yoga teaches you how to get outside of your comfort zone and move beyond your physical and mental boundaries. All the strength, power, freedom and release you discover in each pose you can then take off the yoga mat and use in your everyday life.

Having been around over 5000 years, the power of yoga is evidenced in its longevity. There is also a lot of research on the benefits of yoga and the way it not only reduces the feelings of anxiety and insecurity that many of us experience daily, but that it also changes the neurophysiology of the body by reducing stress hormones and the inflammation that causes fatigue.

What is the difference between yin and yang poses?

The concept of yin and yang comes from Chinese philosophy and represents two complementary principles that interact to maintain harmony. *Thrive Through Yoga* uses a combination of yin and yang poses to create harmony and balance in the bodymind. Yang poses are challenging and dynamic and create strength, while yin poses are passive and relaxing and encourage release. As they challenge our muscles to get stronger, yang poses are held for a shorter amount of time and focus on building physical strength through standing poses, arm balances and backbends. Yin poses are held for a longer period of time and draw our awareness inwards to our breath and our body so we can find emotional balance as well as physical release.

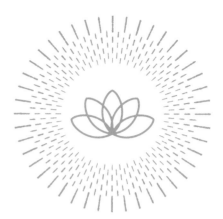

What is the purpose of yoga?

The word 'yoga' comes from the Sanskrit word 'yuj', meaning 'to yolk' or 'to unite'. It is an ancient science which helps those who practise it to find unity between themselves and the world. Despite it often appearing to be about pretzel-like poses, the purpose of yoga runs deeper than what we look like in tree pose or how long we can hold a handstand. With practice, it will give you a sense of peace, wellbeing and connection.

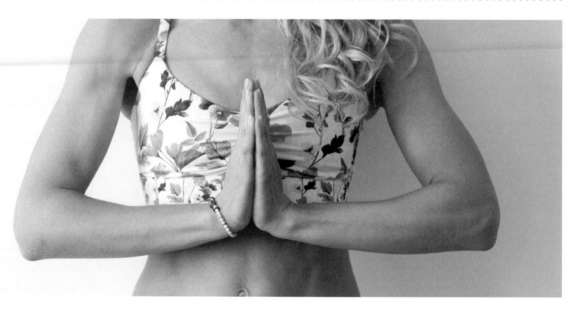

How does yoga encourage thriving?

Yoga is a powerful vehicle for transformation. It facilitates thriving via all five elements that the psychologists Calhoun and Tedeschi identified in their research on post-traumatic growth (PTG). Yoga opens our eyes to a new, more compassionate, heart-centred path, and it gives us a fresh way to relate to others through our physical body. It increases our physical strength through poses and our emotional and psychological resilience through meditation. It also initiates spiritual changes and fosters a greater appreciation for our body, our relationships and our life – all elements of PTG. Recent research has also found that we hold pain in the body leading us to see it as the enemy, so yoga allows us to have empowering body-based experiences which can replace negative views of the body as a source of pain, fear or shame. The limitless possibility for growth on the yoga mat also empowers us to embark on a bigger journey of never-ending growth, transformation and becoming.

2 – Meditation

Meditation is like a cup of coffee for the soul. It's like giving yourself a hug and getting in touch with who you are without all the thoughts and worries and anxieties. It's like a mental gym for you to build the powerful muscles of compassion, understanding and kindness.

Meditation is about transforming the mind so you can live with greater peace and positivity. It has been used for personal growth in India and China since 1500BC, and modern science is starting to recognise its benefits on a physical, mental and emotional level.

Physical benefits of meditation include the way it improves our immunity and increases our energy as well as reducing inflammation, helping to prevent arthritis and asthma, and reducing risk of Alzheimer's and high blood pressure. Improvements in focus, memory and decision making are among some of the mental benefits. Reducing worry and anxiety, decreasing stress and depression, and increasing resilience, optimism and self-esteem are just some of the ways research has found that meditation helps us emotionally.

3 – Psychology and spirituality

Although my professional background is based in the sciences (I studied a degree in psychology and completed a Master's degree in sport and exercise psychology), I have found that the most effective practices for healing combine both spirituality and science.

Psychology is the scientific study of the human mind, and it is an evidence-based practice. This means that the theories and methods used have been researched to see if they are effective. Psychological therapies such as CBT, Dialectical Behaviour Therapy (DBT) and psychotherapy are often used to treat anxiety, stress, depression, eating disorders and other mental health issues.

Spirituality complements psychological methods by expanding healing approaches beyond what can be measured by science. While spiritual methods take some techniques from religions like Buddhism and Taoism, spirituality is not aligned to any religion. Instead, it is about the process of personal transformation so we can own our worth and find meaning in our lives. It is a way of loving and connecting to the world with an open heart and mind.

4 – Ayurveda

Ayurveda is the science of self-healing. It originated in India over 5000 years ago and has recently increased in popularity in the West because of its health benefits.

By making simple diet and lifestyle changes, Ayurveda promotes health, happiness and personal growth by balancing energies in the body. By understanding our own unique make-up, we can empower ourselves as individuals and live a balanced and fulfilled life. As we tune into ourselves and how we feel we can discover who we truly are and create a lifestyle that allows our health to flourish.

One of the things I find really powerful about Ayurveda is that it encourages each of us to take responsibility for our own healing. Rather than seeing ourselves as broken and in need of someone or something external to fix us, it empowers us to look within ourselves for clues as to what really matters and take simple actions for self-healing, wholeness and growth.

The principles of *Thrive Through Yoga*

As well as using modern therapeutic techniques for thriving, I have included many traditional yoga-based healing principles and methods in *Thrive Through Yoga*. These principles have helped people to heal and grow for thousands of years and have been invaluable to me on my own journey.

Although nowadays we think of yoga as a collection of poses, the true aim of yoga is to create unity between our body, mind and spirit (or consciousness) so we can live healthy and fulfilled lives. As well as the poses (traditionally called asanas), there are several other branches of yoga including the yamas and niyamas, which originate in the Yoga Sutras. These are ancient Indian texts containing yogic teachings and philosophies which act as a blueprint for personal growth.

Yamas – Guidelines for wellbeing

The yamas provide us with five guiding principles showing us ways in which we can overcome struggles and expand our lives. I have found them incredibly helpful in easing stress and anxiety because of the way they offer direction on how to relate to others so we can all live life with greater compassion, generosity and peace.

Ahimsa – *Compassion for all living things*

Ahimsa is often translated as *'non-violence'* or *'non-harm'.* It gives us the opportunity to let go of anger, fear or anxiety, and instead make room for peace and calm. This means showing kindness and compassion to ourselves and others through both our thoughts and our actions.

Satya – *Truthfulness*

Being truthful is the bedrock of any healthy relationship – with ourselves, with others and with the world. Whether it's how much coffee we drink or how much our anxiety is holding us back, satya is about being honest with ourselves so we can make the changes needed for healing and growth.

Asteya – *Non-stealing*

The need to steal arises because of a sense of lacking something. When we lack the faith in ourselves that we can create what we need, we look for something to fill that emptiness. When we feel insecure or incomplete, we end up wanting what others have. This could be material things, or it could be that we steal their time by being late or their energy by complaining to them or dwelling on the negative.

The key to cultivating non-stealing is living in abundance – knowing that we have enough and we are enough.

Brahmacharya – *Wise use of energy*

Many of us waste a lot of energy worrying, people pleasing or endlessly pushing ourselves to work harder, get thinner or earn more. In order to be the best version of ourselves we need to understand where we are directing our energy, and whether it is helping us or hurting us so that we can focus our energy towards finding peace and happiness within ourselves.

Aparigrapha – *Non-attachment*

Aparigrapha is all about freedom. This includes freedom from material possessions, negative relationships and stress and anxiety. It teaches us to declutter our minds and our lives by only taking what we need, only keeping what nourishes us, and letting go of anything else. So often we don't follow our dreams because we are too attached to the outcome and worry it won't be good enough. Aparigrapha also gives us the freedom to put our hearts on the line and share ourselves with the world by forgetting about the outcome and simply doing what we love.

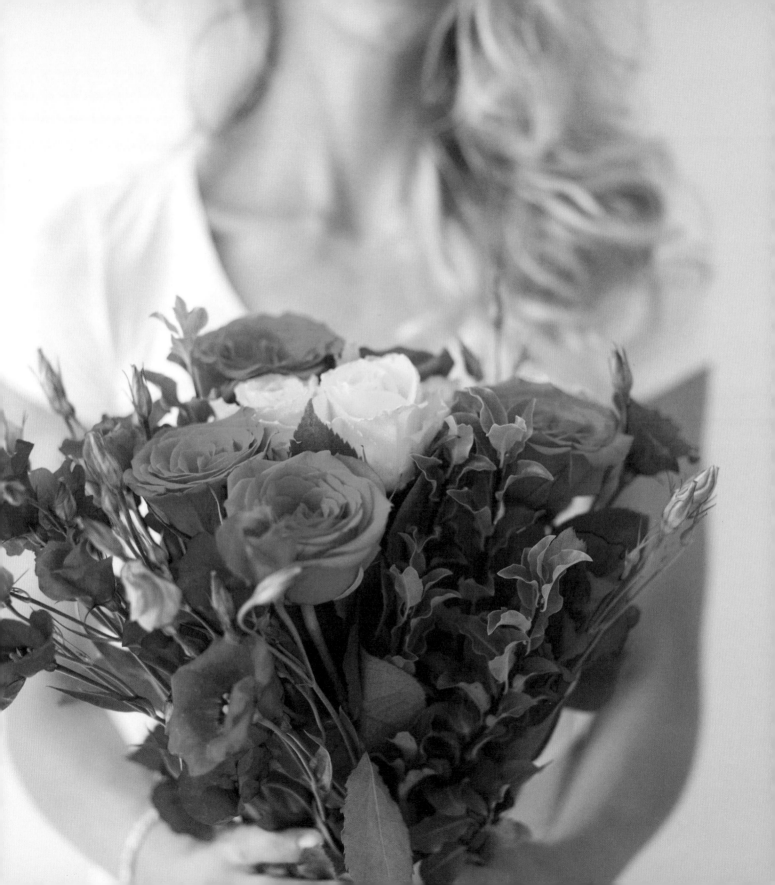

Niyamas – Practices for personal growth

The Niyamas are habits for healthy living which can help make us and the world around us a better place. They focus on creating a more positive and loving relationship with ourselves so that we can create deeper and more meaningful relationships with others.

Saucha – *Purity*

Many of us have destructive or impure habits that don't nourish us. Saucha is about sifting through these habits so everything we do helps us in becoming healthier and happier. It is about having the self-respect to maintain our physical and mental health – decluttering our environment from possessions, wearing clean clothes, bathing or showering daily, eating healthy food, stopping self-criticism and generally getting rid of the disorder in our lives.

Santosha – *Contentment*

Life will throw whatever it wants at us, so santosha is about being happy with who we are and what we have. This doesn't mean we can't grow or work towards goals, it just means we need to recognise which goals are really important to our wellbeing and work towards them without basing our sense of peace and joy on achieving them. In order to escape the cycle of happiness, sadness, calmness, anxiety, love and fear, we need to find happiness and love within ourselves so we can love, trust and give ourselves fully to the world.

Tapas – *Self-discipline*

Tapas is our inner fire. It's what gets our heart pumping and gives us the courage to get outside of our comfort zone so we can heal and grow. It is the burning desire to learn and do the work required to find a place of peace and freedom. This involves having the determination to follow a healthy diet and exercise regularly, to break unhealthy habits such as smoking or drinking, to ignore the voices in our head that tell us we're not good enough, and to refrain from any actions that cause us suffering or prevent us from thriving.

Svadhyaya – *Self-study*

By studying ourselves we become more aware of the things that hurt us or cause us harm and of those that heal us and make us happy. Svadhyaya encourages us to question our thoughts, feelings and actions: Why am I feeling stressed? Why am I drinking this cup of coffee? Why am I thinking about the size of my thighs? It helps us to be fully aware, to recognise habits and thought processes that are harming us, and to notice what we are doing and how we are feeling from moment to moment. This self-observation often acts as a catalyst for healing and transformation.

Ishvara pranidhana –
Commitment to connection

Ishvara pranidhana is about our connection to something bigger than ourselves. This may be a God, a universal power, all of humanity or a sense that we are all one. It's about putting our selfish desires and comforts aside and doing what is best for humanity. Instead of being ruled by our ego, it's about surrendering the control, worries, judgements and fears, trusting our intuition and doing our best for the world. This will ultimately lead to freedom.

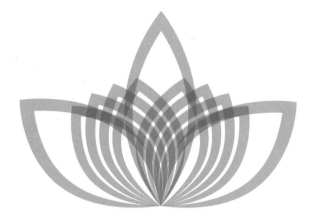

Chakras – Energy centres

The chakras are the energy centres of the body which, when balanced, create a sense of peace and wellbeing. They were first mentioned in ancient Indian texts over 2500 years ago and over recent years scientists and biologists have theorised that these energy centres correspond to areas of the brain, nervous system and endocrine system. It is helpful to work with the chakras because we can identify any blockages of energy or emotion that might be causing struggles and then we can work to clear any blockages so our energy can flow freely once more.

Muladhara – *Root chakra*

Located at the base of the spine, the root chakra is the centre of stability and security. When this chakra is closed we struggle with money and food. When it is open, we feel grounded, safe and fearless.

Svadisthana – *Sacral chakra*

The sacral chakra is located just below the belly button and is the centre of creativity and sexuality. When this chakra is imbalanced we can feel emotionally unstable and struggle with depression and addiction. When it is balanced we feel pleasure, joy and a sense of abundance.

Manipura – *Solar plexus chakra*

Located in the upper abdomen, the solar plexus chakra is our source of personal power. When it is closed or out of balance we suffer from lack of self-worth and low self-esteem, but when it is balanced we feel confident and have a strong sense of purpose in our lives.

Anahata – *Heart chakra*

The heart chakra links the first three physical chakras (root, sacral and solar plexus) with the upper chakras of the spirit. It is our ability to love, so when it is out of balance and our heart is closed, we can feel anger, jealousy, fear and hatred towards ourselves and others. When it is open and love is flowing freely, we feel love, compassion and connection.

Vishudda – *Throat chakra*

The throat chakra is our centre of expression and communication. When it is out of balance we may struggle with social anxiety and have difficulty expressing our feelings. When it is balanced we feel confident in expressing our wants and needs.

Ajna – *Third eye chakra*

Ajna chakra is located between the eyebrows and is the centre for intuition. When it is blocked we may suffer from confusion, indecisiveness and a lack of trust in ourselves. When it is balanced we feel imaginative, are confident in listening to our gut instincts and can make decisions that nourish us.

Sahasrara – *Crown chakra*

Located on the top of the head, the crown chakra is the centre of enlightenment and connection – with ourselves, with others and with the universe. When it is blocked or out of balance we can feel lonely and disconnected, and we may feel a lack of direction in our lives. When it is balanced we feel beauty within us and all around us, we feel connection with ourselves and the world and we have a sense of pure bliss.

What is energy?

Throughout the *Thrive Through Yoga* journey we explore how to release physical and mental stress, toxins and anything else that blocks our flow of energy. The energy being referred to is commonly known as bio-energy, subtle energy, chi, or prana, and encompasses all forms of energy (e.g. nutrition, sun, oxygen, thoughts and emotions). Recent research has found that energy practices promote optimal health through stress reduction as shown by their positive effects on heart rate, inflammation and telomere length (a biological marker for longevity and healthy ageing).

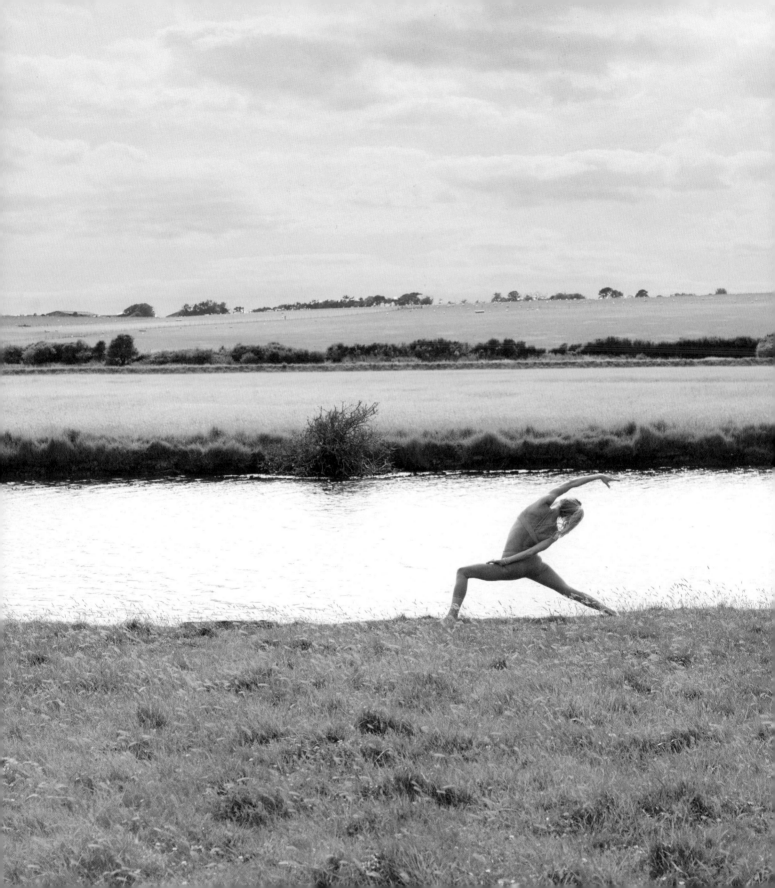

Part 2:
The Thrive Sequence

The Thrive Sequence is the foundation of your yoga practice throughout your *Thrive Through Yoga* journey. It's a 10-minute sequence you will be guided through daily as part of the yoga routine you are given on each new day.

It is a flowing, breath-synchronized sequence traditionally called a vinyasa, meaning you match each movement to your breath. As you begin to work with your breath like this you'll discover how everything you do can be a moving meditation – taking you away from any stress, anxiety or fear and bringing you into the present moment. It's important you do this sequence daily if possible to keep your inner fire ignited so you can continue on the journey of self-discovery and transformation.

The Thrive Sequence also has many other physical, emotional and energetic benefits, including warming and awakening the body by softening the muscles, opening the joints and stimulating circulation. It will help you to build a stronger and more flexible body, relax the nervous system, release tension and get rid of toxins. You will begin to feel what is happening in your body and discover more openness, more balanced energy and a more open heart.

One of the main things I've learnt on my own journey is that not everything worthwhile has to be hard or involve blood, sweat and tears. The Thrive Sequence will also teach you to move along the path of least resistance and live with effortless effort, so you can stay balanced amid the constant changes in your life. As you practise the sequence it's important to remember that yoga isn't about achieving anything. It's about practice and patience. There is no end to what you can learn, how much you can grow, or how deeply you can love yourself.

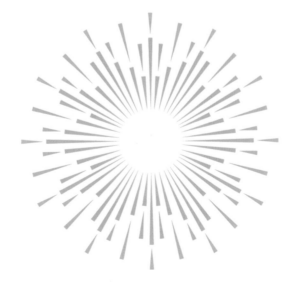

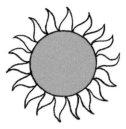

The Thrive Sequence

Whether you're an experienced yogi or a complete yoga novice, you can practise the Thrive Sequence confidently and compassionately by working with your body. Be mindful of how you feel each time you practise the sequence and move with awareness, remembering that yoga is about practice not perfection. Descriptions of all poses and variations are in the Yoga Pose Library in Part 6 of the book (see pages 131–185), and you can watch a video of the full sequence at www.NicolaJaneHobbs.com.

Start at the front of your mat, standing with your toes, ankles and knees together and bring your palms to your heart for **Mountain**.

As you inhale, raise your hands above your head into **Upward Salute** and as you exhale dive forwards to bring your fingertips to the floor, for **Standing Forward Bend**.

On your next inhale, lift and lengthen your chest forwards so your spine is parallel to the floor into **Lift and Lengthen**.

As you exhale step or jump back to **Plank** pose and lower yourself either all the way down to the floor, or see if you can hover just above it in **Crocodile** pose.

On your next inhale, lift your chest to **Up Dog**, and as you exhale lift your hips up and back to **Down Dog**.

As you inhale lift your right leg to the sky to **Three Legged Dog**, and as you exhale step your right foot forwards between your hands for **Warrior Prep**.

On your next inhale lift your hands to the sky to **Warrior 1**.

Exhale and open your hips out so they are facing the long edge of your mat, at the same time as spreading your arms out wide to **Warrior 2**.

Inhale and lean back to **Reverse Warrior**, so you are reaching your left arm down your left leg.

Exhale and bring your arms forwards to rest your right fingertips on the inside of your right foot, and shoot your left arm up and over into **Side Angle**.

Inhale and lean back to **Reverse Warrior**, and then as you exhale windmill both arms forwards to bring one hand either side of your right foot into **Warrior Prep**.

Inhale and step back to **Plank**. Exhale and lower down to **Crocodile**.

Inhale to **Up Dog** and exhale to **Down Dog**.

On your next inhale, repeat the flow on your left side.

In yoga we practise poses on the right side first because it is associated with more active, warming energy whereas the left side is associated with calming, cooling energy. This means we can energise our body and mind using the right side and then calm it down by practising the pose on the left side. By always starting on the right side we also ensure we practise both sides instead of getting confused as to which side we did a pose on first.

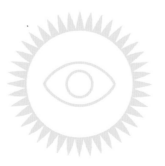

The Thrive Sequence

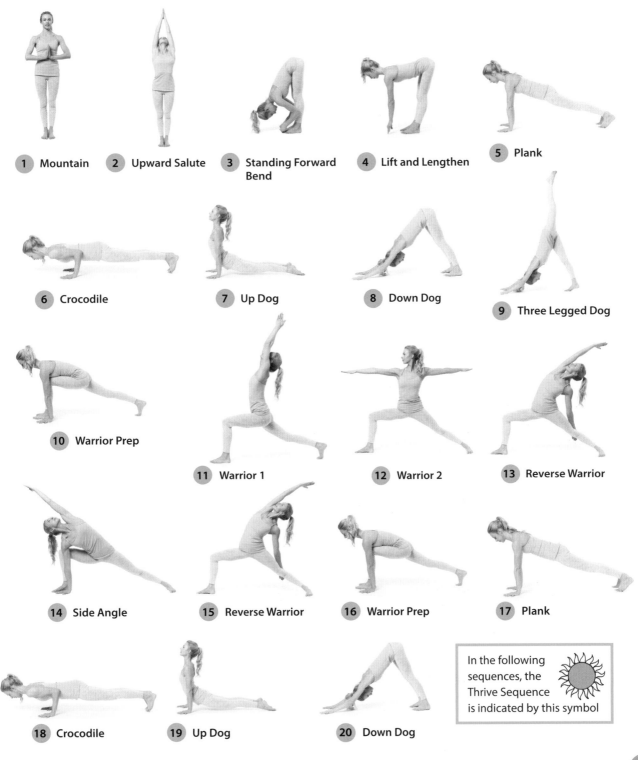

1 Mountain

2 Upward Salute

3 Standing Forward Bend

4 Lift and Lengthen

5 Plank

6 Crocodile

7 Up Dog

8 Down Dog

9 Three Legged Dog

10 Warrior Prep

11 Warrior 1

12 Warrior 2

13 Reverse Warrior

14 Side Angle

15 Reverse Warrior

16 Warrior Prep

17 Plank

18 Crocodile

19 Up Dog

20 Down Dog

In the following sequences, the Thrive Sequence is indicated by this symbol

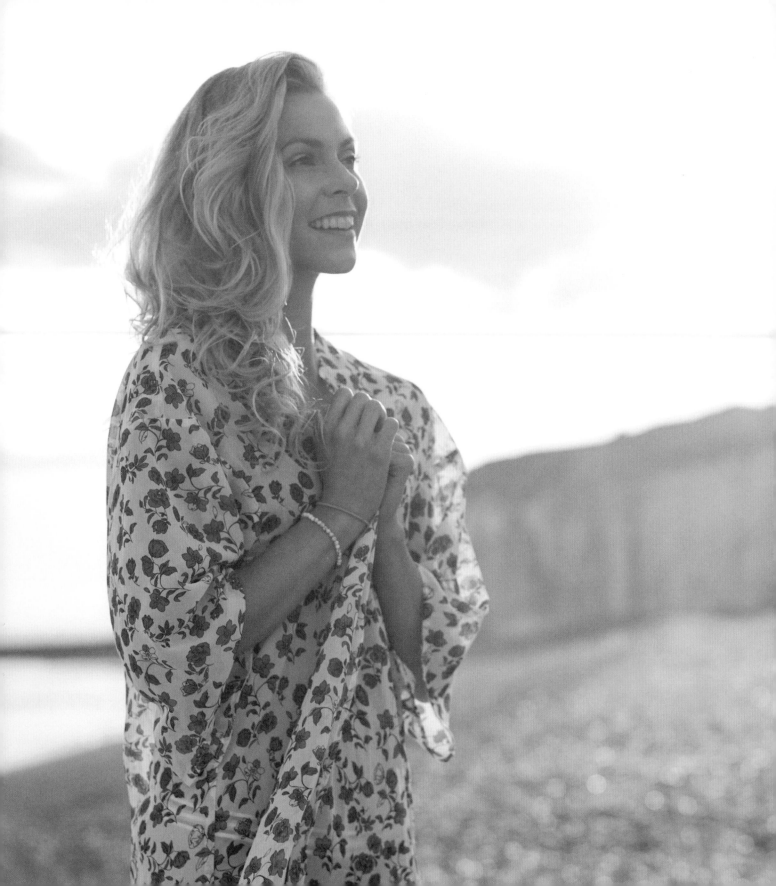

Part 3: The Journey

Imagine yourself as a little plot of earth. At the moment, it might be full of rocks and weeds from the stresses and anxieties in your life but, as you go on this journey, I want you to start tending to it. Flowers won't suddenly appear overnight, but with the tools this book gives you, you will build the faith and confidence that something beautiful will grow. As long as you do not give up on yourself and you keep cultivating your little plot of earth patiently, you will learn how to nourish yourself, how to love yourself, and how to thrive.

Each day, you will be introduced to a new theme to focus on and help you grow. As well as the Thrive Sequence, you will be given specific yoga poses that relate to the theme and the relevant chakras and energy pathways. It doesn't matter if you find some of the poses difficult, or struggle to concentrate. It doesn't matter if you step on your yoga mat with a jumbled mind and a heavy heart. It doesn't matter if you're feeling on top of the world or if you've had a rough day. All that matters is that you show up and do your best in every practice.

Intention Setting

Before you begin your yoga practice, as you start to connect to your breath, set an intention that ties in with the theme for the day. For example, Day 1 of the journey is about self-awareness, so your intention could be to become more aware of how your body feels, or notice what mental chatter is going through your head as you practise.

You will also be given a mantra or meditation technique to quieten your mind and a heart-centred exploration for personal growth which encourages you to get out of your head so you can follow your heart.

Before you begin…

In order to fully embrace the *Thrive Through Yoga* journey you need to set aside 30–60 minutes a day to practise the yoga sequences and meditations, and give yourself the time for each heart-centred exploration. You can spread this throughout the day if it's easier for you (for example 25 minutes in the morning for the yoga routine and meditation, and 15 minutes in the evening for the heart-centred exploration). If you are struggling to find the time, then be aware of how long you spend mindlessly watching TV or flicking through social media. You may find that you do have the time available, you just need to rearrange how you use it – so use this time for your daily *Thrive Through Yoga* practice. It might be helpful to practise at the same time in the same place every day: block it out in your diary and tell your family or housemates about it so you are not disturbed.

You might also find it helpful to get yourself a yoga mat, block, strap and few candles to create a calming space for you to practise your yoga routines and meditations, as well as a notebook to keep all your heart-centred explorations in one place. You don't need to wear anything special when practising the yoga routines – just clothing that is comfortable and allows you to move freely.

If you have any concerns or questions about beginning your journey please feel free to contact me via www.NicolaJaneHobbs.com or on social media at @NicolaJaneHobbs.

Day 1: Self-Awareness

Knowing ourselves is the beginning of all transformation. Of ourselves. Of our relationships. Of our world.

This is the part where you find out who you are. The part where you stop judging yourself. Where you take off your mask and get out of your own way.

Most of us don't know ourselves to our fullest capacity. We are all great at acting and putting on a show that everything is perfectly fine because we are afraid that showing our fears, or shame, or vulnerability means we are weak. But being aware of these feelings, however painful they may be, and moving gently towards whatever scares us instead of running away is the first step to thriving.

But before we begin, I want to gently warn you that self-awareness can be messy and confusing. Learning about yourself is a wild ride of healing, helplessness, chaos, clarity and awakening.

I started truly learning about myself eight years ago. After spending most of my teenage years in self-destruct mode, I hit rock bottom. In that moment of desperation and despair I realised that throughout all the years of therapy and treatment, I had been looking outside of myself for someone to tell me what to do, to save me, to fix me. I felt like doctors, therapists, friends and family didn't understand me or know what was best and, because they were supposedly the experts and even they couldn't make me better, I would be trapped in a world of anxiety and sadness forever. But they weren't the experts, I was the expert. And as soon as I grasped this, I began the journey of learning about who I was, who I wanted to be, what my weaknesses were, and what I needed to let go of to be truly happy.

Self-awareness is about having a clear understanding of who we are – our personality, thoughts, emotions, beliefs, strengths, weaknesses, passions and motivations. It includes:

- *Understanding our emotions, what triggers them and how we can use them most effectively.*
- *Noticing negative thought patterns such as being overly self-critical, beating ourselves up over how we look, or undermining our abilities.*
- *Recognising destructive behaviours and habits including using food, alcohol or drugs to numb our emotions, over-exercising and overworking.*
- *Tuning into our body so that we can access our intuition.*
- *Becoming honest with ourselves about what we want, what is holding us back, and where we can grow.*
- *Accepting that we are responsible for our actions and the direction of our life.*

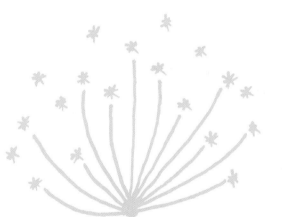

Self-awareness is crucial for the simple reason that you cannot love someone you don't know. Only when you are self-aware, do you have the ability to genuinely love yourself. And because you love yourself, you can be the real you. No mask. No armour. The raw, real, imperfectly perfect you.

Heart-Centred Exploration

Today's exploration is simple: People watching. Find somewhere to sit like a coffee shop or a park bench and just watch. As you watch, notice what you are thinking and feeling. Many people find that rather than watching with complete openness, they will be judging, criticizing and sizing up everyone who passes. Normally when we judge others it is an extension of the way we judge ourselves but this self-judgement has become so ingrained that we aren't even aware that we are doing it. It can be quite shocking to become aware of how critical and mean we can be about ourselves and others so treat this exploration of awareness as a revelation for the rest of your journey.

Self-Awareness Sequence

One of the first steps to self-awareness is through the body. Today's sequence is about tuning into your body and getting to know yourself better through some basic poses which focus on the grounding nature of the root chakra. Remember that detailed instructions for all poses are in the Yoga Pose Library in Part 6 of the book (see pages 131–185).

Some of the poses are held for a certain number of breaths and some for minutes. Before you begin, count how many breaths you take in a minute at rest (usually between 12 and 20) and then if you find yourself getting distracted by clock watching you can count your breaths instead. For example, if you do 15 breaths a minute and you want to hold the pose for 2 minutes, instead of setting a stopwatch or watching the clock, you can do 30 breaths.

Each *Thrive Through Yoga* sequence begins with your intention setting, or sankalpa in Sanskrit (see page 31). This is your brief, positive statement honouring something or someone in the course of your practice. The purpose of your sankalpa is to provide an anchor for your practice and to help you live less from habit and more from intention.

Breath Awareness Meditation

In general, we tend to practise meditation after we have practised yoga so any stress has already been released from our body. If the body is relaxed, it is much easier for us to be still and calm our mind.

In today's meditation we simply focus on our breath. As we increase our awareness of the breath, we increase our awareness of our true self – no ego, no thoughts and no anxiety.

Begin by finding a comfortable seated position and close your eyes. Take a couple of moments to simply be and notice any thoughts, feelings and physical sensations, without doing anything about them. Now bring your awareness to your breath. Notice it as it moves in and out automatically and effortlessly. Your mind will wander away from your breath to begin with, so when it does, just bring your awareness back to your breathing – letting any thoughts and feelings come and go.

Stay focused on your breath in this meditation for just five minutes today and, if you want to, build up how long you meditate for over time.

Day 1: Self-Awareness Sequence

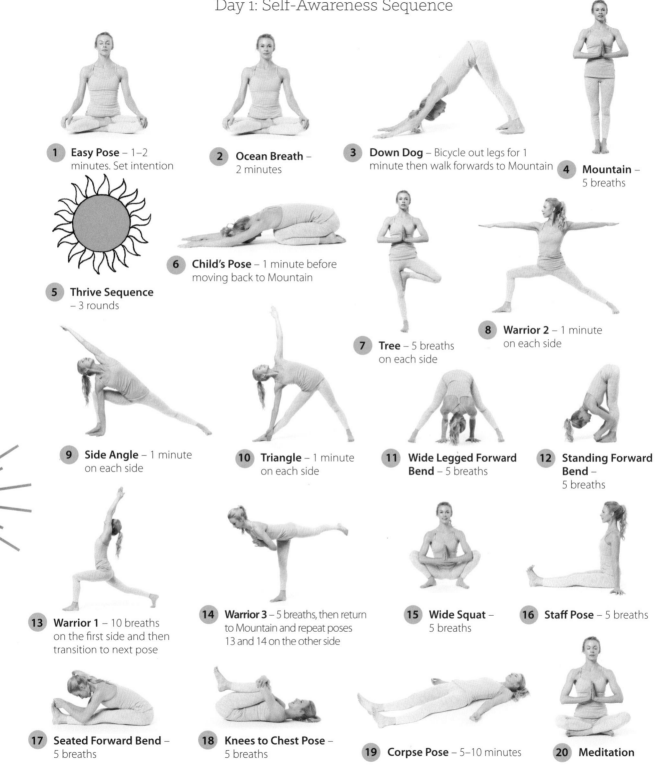

1. **Easy Pose** – 1–2 minutes. Set intention

2. **Ocean Breath** – 2 minutes

3. **Down Dog** – Bicycle out legs for 1 minute then walk forwards to Mountain

4. **Mountain** – 5 breaths

5. **Thrive Sequence** – 3 rounds

6. **Child's Pose** – 1 minute before moving back to Mountain

7. **Tree** – 5 breaths on each side

8. **Warrior 2** – 1 minute on each side

9. **Side Angle** – 1 minute on each side

10. **Triangle** – 1 minute on each side

11. **Wide Legged Forward Bend** – 5 breaths

12. **Standing Forward Bend** – 5 breaths

13. **Warrior 1** – 10 breaths on the first side and then transition to next pose

14. **Warrior 3** – 5 breaths, then return to Mountain and repeat poses 13 and 14 on the other side

15. **Wide Squat** – 5 breaths

16. **Staff Pose** – 5 breaths

17. **Seated Forward Bend** – 5 breaths

18. **Knees to Chest Pose** – 5 breaths

19. **Corpse Pose** – 5–10 minutes

20. **Meditation**

Day 2: Slowing Down and Being Present

Lose yourself in the here and now. That is where you will find freedom. That is where you will find yourself.

The world moves pretty fast and it's easy to lose ourselves in the chaos. Many of us live our lives in an anxious struggle of multi-tasking, achieving goals, meeting expectations and getting through our to-do lists, so it's easy to lose awareness of the present moment. We think too much, we want too much, we worry too much and we forget how blissful it feels to just be.

Society doesn't make it easy for us to slow down and be present either. It has an incredible power to create dissatisfaction and desire in such a way that, in order to be happy, we need to have this or do that. It's as if we can never enjoy ourselves where we are or with what we have, so we anxiously rush through life trying to do more, have more, be more.

But the faster we live the less we notice the good things in our lives, the less we are able to listen to what our body is telling us, and the more we end up struggling with anxiety, tension, stress and worry. This is why slowing down and being present is so important on our journey.

One of the biggest discoveries I made on my own journey is that suffering needs time. When you are present no fear or stress can survive in you. When I was having a bad day this helped me to be with the anxiety or the depression without fearing that it would be that way forever.

Slowing down and being present is about breaking the habit of busy-ness and living a more mindful, intentional and compassionate life. It includes:

- Paying attention to whatever is happening in our lives without judgement.
- Being aware of what we are thinking and doing.
- Being with the present experience instead of going on autopilot.
- Not clinging to or rejecting the present moment.
- Being fully with the people we are sharing time with.
- Slowing down our breathing, speaking, walking and eating.
- Responding to life's pressures calmly and mindfully.

Slowing down and being present is important because it gives us the time to get to know ourselves better and truly see the things that matter most. Much research is being done on the benefits of mindfulness on physical, mental and emotional wellbeing, and it has been found to decrease anxiety, stress, depression and exhaustion, reduce addiction and self-destructive behaviour and improve immunity, circulation, self-awareness and emotional resilience.

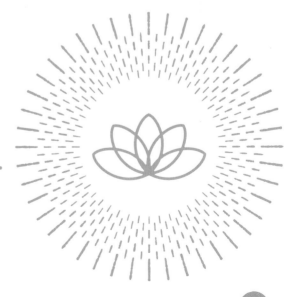

Heart-Centred Exploration

The present moment is the key to all transformation, so being present while we're doing the simple things in life will help us stay present in times of stress and struggle. For today's exploration we are going to involve all five senses to help us stay present.

Start off by making yourself a cup of tea or get yourself a glass of juice and find a quiet place to sit. Begin by noticing the colour of your drink. Is it clear or cloudy? Bright or dull? Then, as you hold the cup or glass, notice the temperature. Does it warm your hands or cool them? Take a sniff of your drink and see what it smells like. Is it delicate or overpowering? Then take a big slurp and notice the sound it makes. Take another sip and tune into the taste. Is it sweet? Sour? Bitter? Spend five minutes enjoying your tea or juice, using your five senses to keep you grounded in the present moment. Notice the calmness you experience by slowing down and focusing only on what is happening right now.

Slowing Down Sequence

For the slowing down sequence we'll be practising a type of yoga called yin yoga. This style brings balance to our fast-paced lives by encouraging us to hold poses for two to five minutes each. If you find your mind wandering or you start to wriggle, then bring your awareness to your breath – being aware of your breath gently forces you into the present moment.

Remember to begin by setting your intention, or sankalpa in Sanskrit (see page 31). This is something or someone you would like to dedicate your practice to, to help you focus and bring meaning to each pose.

Present Moment Meditation

The present moment meditation is a wonderful tool to use anytime you are feeling anxious, stressed or depressed. It helps to relax us by shifting our awareness from the past or the future and bringing it to right now. When we first start meditating, it's easy for our mind to wander so in this meditation we give it simple things to focus on. Read the instructions first and come back to them throughout the meditation if you need to. You can also listen to some of the meditations in the *Thrive Through Yoga* journey at www.NicolaJaneHobbs.com.

Start off by finding a comfortable seated position either on the floor or on a chair or sofa. Close your eyes and take a couple of deep breaths.

Begin by focusing on any sounds around you – start off with the most obvious and bring your awareness to subtler sounds like the quiet ticking of a clock or distant birdsong. Move from sound to sound, just allowing them to wash over you as they pass.

After a minute, bring your awareness to your body. Feel your bottom sitting on the floor or on the chair. Feel your clothes on your skin and your hands resting. Tune into any tension you're holding in your jaw or shoulders, any fluttering in your stomach, or any pain in your body. Notice any feelings – stress, anxiety, worry, and watch how they shift and change without getting involved in them or trying to identify where they're from. Allow them to pass and stay present with any other feelings that arise.

Now bring your awareness to your thoughts and, without feeling like you have to act on them, let them go. It can help to visualise these thoughts as clouds and your mind as the sky – visualise the clouds passing until you have a clear blue sky and your mind is clear and calm.

Now bring your awareness back to your breath. Don't try and control it, just notice how it becomes slower and deeper the more relaxed you become. Stay here for a couple of minutes until you are ready to open your eyes.

Day 2: Slowing Down Sequence

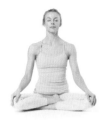

1 **Easy Pose** – 1–2 minutes. Set intention

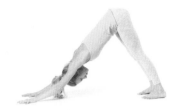

2 **Down Dog** – Bicycle out legs for 1 minute then walk forwards to Mountain

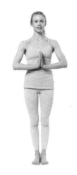

3 **Mountain** – 5 breaths

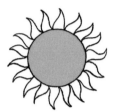

4 **Thrive Sequence** – 3 rounds

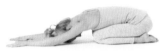

5 **Child's Pose** – 1 minute

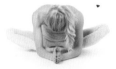

6 **Butterfly** – 3 minutes

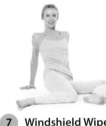

7 **Windshield Wipers** – 10 times

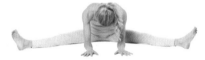

8 **Straddle** – 3 minutes

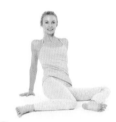

9 **Windshield Wipers** – 10 times

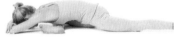

10 **Sleeping Pigeon** – 2 minutes each side. Stretch out in Down Dog in between sides

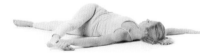

11 **Reclining Twist** – 2 minutes each side

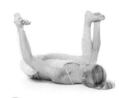

12 **Happy Baby** – 2 minutes

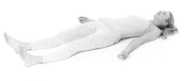

13 **Corpse Pose** – 5–10 minutes

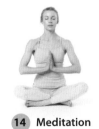

14 **Meditation**

Day 3: Forgiveness and Letting Go

Let it hurt. Let it heal. Let it go.

Sometimes life feels heavy. That's because we all walk around with baggage. But when we take a moment to look inside our bags we often discover that much of what we are carrying we no longer need. We might be carrying around guilt or shame over past mistakes, habits and behaviours that no longer nourish us, or an idea in our head of what our life should be like.

So today is about discovering that you don't have to carry any unnecessary and unnourishing baggage with you any more. It's about forgiving yourself so you can heal. It's about loving yourself enough to let go of what no longer serves you and creating space for something better.

Forgiveness brings peace. And the main person we need to forgive is usually ourselves. We are all human. We make mistakes. We do things we aren't proud of. But don't let shame and sadness run your life.

A big part of forgiveness is letting go. It may be letting go of shame or guilt, letting go of self-critical thoughts and self-destructive behaviours, or letting go of parts of your lifestyle such as a job that makes you unhappy, a diet that makes you feel trapped or an unhealthy relationship – with food, drink, social media, a friend or a partner.

It took me a long time to forgive myself and let go. I tried to recover from anorexia so many times while still being at war with myself and carrying the guilt and shame of the disorder. Only when I realised that we have to forgive ourselves before we can fix ourselves did I begin to heal. Another thing I've learnt is that forgiveness is not a one-time thing. It's something you have to do every day, over and over again – as many times as it takes to find freedom.

Forgiveness and letting go isn't about pretending something didn't happen or that it doesn't hurt. It's about understanding the lessons we can learn from the experience without holding onto the pain. It involves:

· Releasing negative thoughts of bitterness and resentment.

· Freeing ourselves from pain and anger that has built up over time.

· Acknowledging our own inner pain and expressing it in ways that will not hurt ourselves or others.

· Choosing to move our focus from past hurt to the present moment.

· Facing up to the emotional barriers of fear and anger that are causing us to hold onto feelings, behaviours, people or things which are harming us.

· Cultivating non-attachment. For example, working towards goals without thinking we need to accomplish them to be happy, being in a relationship while letting the other person be free, or starting a weight-loss regime without believing we need to be a certain weight to love our body.

Letting go and forgiving ourselves is a decision. It means saying, 'I've felt ashamed, scared and angry long enough. I am releasing my shame, fear and anger because I don't need to carry them any more'. Once we are no longer beating ourselves up for our mistakes, we can learn to love ourselves in healthy ways and realise we have value and worth.

Heart-Centred Exploration

Today's exploration focuses on forgiving yourself by writing yourself a letter.

Before you can let go of any emotion you have to feel it fully. The emotion could be anything from feeling shame about your body, guilt for not meeting your parents' expectations, regret for hurting someone you love or any other emotion that is holding you back.

Begin by writing down the emotion, event or experience that you would like to let go of and forgive yourself for. Write in as much detail as you can. Allow yourself to feel the hurt and ask yourself how long you have held onto these feelings for and how much they affect your everyday life. If you need to, discuss how you feel with someone close to you and they can help you to realise that we all make mistakes which are in need of forgiveness and that you don't deserve to feel pain or hurt.

Once you have given yourself a bit of time to grieve the feelings, shred or burn the piece of paper you wrote your emotions down on as a visual symbol of letting go. If you need to, repeat this with other areas of your life where you are in need of forgiveness so that you can move on and live with greater freedom. If the hurt, shame or anger are triggered again at some point in your life, gently remind yourself that you have forgiven yourself and chosen to move on so that you can grow.

Letting Go Sequence

Letting go is a yin-like quality. There is no pushing or pulling. We don't have to try to let go. We just have to let go. This can be difficult because letting go isn't valued in our culture but, with practice, you will find peace and power in doing so. Today's sequence consists of yin poses. Holding each pose passively for a longer period of time gives you the chance to focus on your breath. Notice the ease at which you exhale – the effortlessness at which you 'let go' of your breath and see if you can do the same with other sensations in the poses – allow them, label them without judgement, and then let them go.

Forgiveness Meditation

Forgiveness isn't something that can be forced. It only happens when we open our hearts and let go of the hurt. Today's meditation focuses on the way that blame, bitterness and resentment – the opposites of forgiveness – keep us trapped, and how by forgiving ourselves we set ourselves free.

Find a quiet space and awaken the feelings of shame, guilt, anger, regret or any other feeling you want to release. The feeling might be tied to a moment in your life, a memory or a thought. Don't dwell on where the feeling comes from, just focus on the feeling itself. As you do so, take a deep breath and visualise yourself as a bird trapped in a cage – trapped by the shame, guilt, anger or fear. As you breathe out, visualise yourself flying out from the cage and setting yourself free by letting go of the negative feelings and forgiving yourself. Do this as many times as you need to – breathing in the feeling of being a bird trapped in a cage, and breathing out the feeling of setting yourself free.

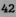

Day 3: Letting Go Sequence

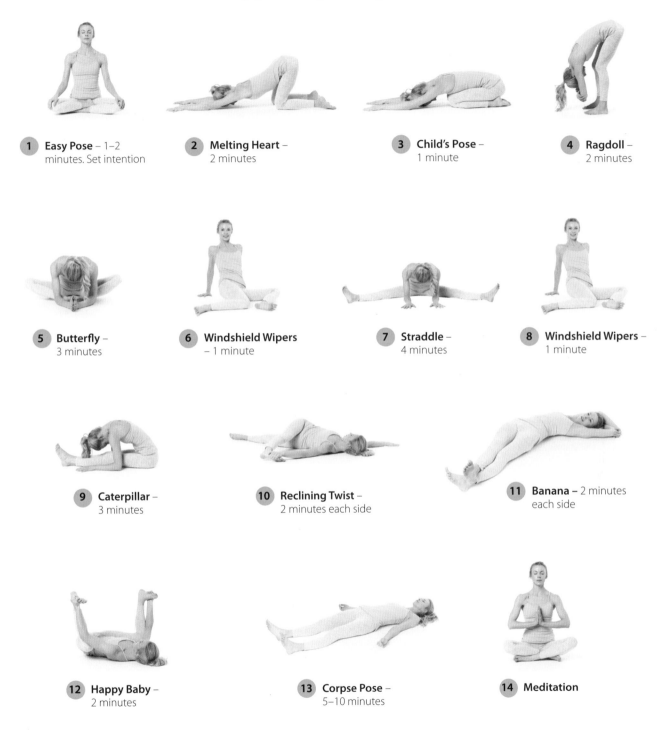

1 **Easy Pose** – 1–2 minutes. Set intention

2 **Melting Heart** – 2 minutes

3 **Child's Pose** – 1 minute

4 **Ragdoll** – 2 minutes

5 **Butterfly** – 3 minutes

6 **Windshield Wipers** – 1 minute

7 **Straddle** – 4 minutes

8 **Windshield Wipers** – 1 minute

9 **Caterpillar** – 3 minutes

10 **Reclining Twist** – 2 minutes each side

11 **Banana** – 2 minutes each side

12 **Happy Baby** – 2 minutes

13 **Corpse Pose** – 5–10 minutes

14 **Meditation**

Day 4: Nourishment and Self-Care

*When you nourish yourself
you radiate light into the world.
And the world needs your light.*

Nourishment is the opposite of neglect. Self-care is the opposite of self-harm. When we nourish and care for ourselves we are making a conscious decision to do what is best for ourselves and our health.

We can neglect ourselves in many ways – eating too much, eating too little, under-exercising, over-exercising, staying in a destructive relationship, working long hours, going to bed late, constantly criticising ourselves. When we neglect ourselves like this we are sending a message that we aren't worth the time to look after. But when we begin to nourish ourselves we swap this message of worthlessness for one of self-love and self-respect that reassures us that we are someone of value whose wellbeing is sacred.

Nourishing ourselves is closely related to letting go. If something in our life is not nourishing our soul, we need to get rid of it in order to make room for those things that do. This might be eating natural foods, walking in nature and spending time with loved ones. Or it might be taking naps, baking a cake or just taking some time to enjoy our own company.

One of the things that stopped me from nourishing myself in the past was that I thought self-care was selfish. But in all honesty, my stressed-out, anxiety-riddled self was no good for anyone. Only when we are so full of nourishment will it overflow into loving others. And when we do start to nourish ourselves, the world takes on a different appearance – food becomes a way to show self-respect instead of being a source of shame and fear, exercise becomes a way to reward our body with strength instead of punishing it for eating too much, and life as a whole becomes a lot kinder and more meaningful.

Another thing that's important to remember is that you are allowed to nourish yourself right now – not when you lose 10 pounds, or get a boyfriend or finish every task on your to-do list. This nourishment looks different for everyone but it involves:

- Any intentional actions we take to care for our physical, mental and emotional health.

- Having the self-worth and self-confidence to look after ourselves.

- Being as gentle with ourselves as we are with other people.

- Asking ourselves what we need and making sure we receive it.

- Getting adequate nutrition, exercise and sleep.

- Not depleting ourselves or sacrificing our own needs.

No matter how we feel, we can control how we treat ourselves. Whether we feel happy and strong, or hopeless and inadequate, the need to nourish ourselves and sow the seeds of our future wellbeing is unconditional.

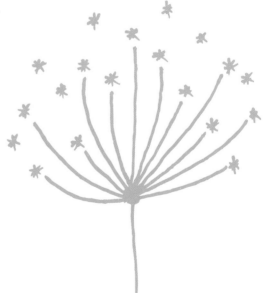

Heart-Centred Exploration

Simply devote today to nourishing yourself more. Life can be pretty noisy and confusing, so it's important we find ways to regularly include a little bit of love and care for ourselves among the busy-ness.

Start off by making a list of things that you enjoy and leave you feeling restored. Some ideas might be: getting outside in nature, spending time with people who make you laugh, taking a break from social media, decluttering, cooking a tasty meal, practising yoga, having a bath or reading a book.

Choose one or two of these things to explore today and notice how you feel afterwards. Once you discover something that nourishes you, make sure you care enough about yourself to make room for it in your life. You can do this by scheduling it into your diary and, whether it's a yoga class, walk in nature or baking session, make sure you prioritise it as much as you would a work meeting or parents' evening. Valuing self-care in this way allows you to restore yourself so you can care for others with the same love and tenderness.

Self-Care Sequence

Yoga is about rewarding your body with strength and openness, so today's sequence focuses on the solar plexus chakra. When this chakra is balanced we live with self-worth, self-care and self-confidence.

Self-Care Meditation

Meditation is one of the best ways to nourish ourselves. Today's meditation is a *'Metta'* meditation – also known as a loving-kindness meditation. This meditation originally comes from Buddhist traditions and is now supported by scientific research for its benefits including: increasing self-care, self-compassion, contentment, hope, gratitude and joy, and decreasing depression, chronic pain, anger, distress and self-criticism.

Begin by finding a comfortable seated position and close your eyes. Start by developing a feeling of loving-kindness towards yourself using an aspiration for nourishment and self-care, such as: *'May I do what is best for me and my health so my fears get weaker and my true self gets stronger.'* You can put this aspiration into your own words to make it more personal to you.

If you find it too difficult to cultivate these feelings towards yourself at first, then you can start cultivating loving-kindness towards someone you love – a child, a parent, even a pet. For example, *'May my Dad do what is best for himself and his health so his fears get weaker and his true self gets stronger.'* Once you cultivate this feeling, see if you can awaken loving-kindness towards yourself. As you deepen this feeling, widen the circle of loving-kindness to:

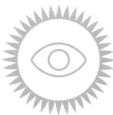

- Someone you love
- A friend
- A stranger or someone neutral
- Someone you find difficult or offensive
- All of the above equally
- All beings

Spend one to two minutes awakening loving-kindness for each of the individuals and groups.

Day 4: Self-Care Sequence

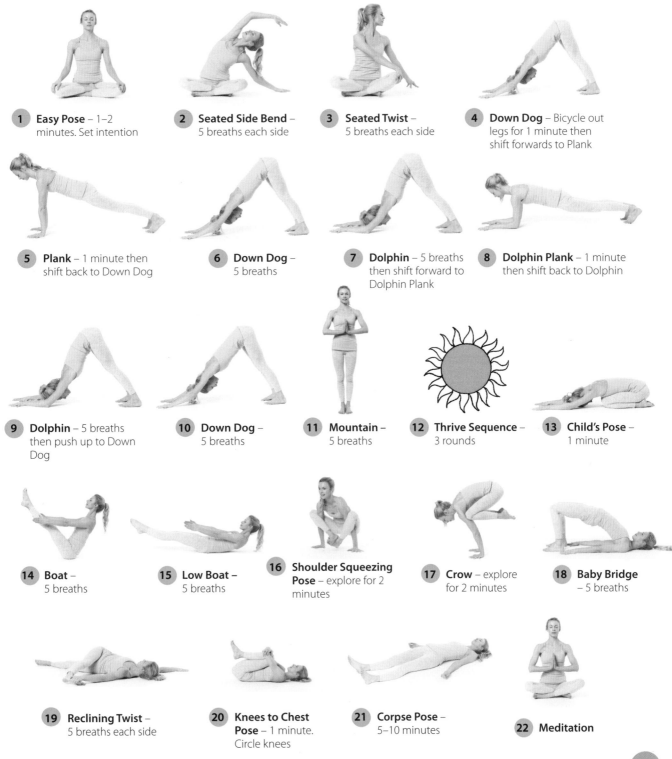

1 **Easy Pose** – 1–2 minutes. Set intention

2 **Seated Side Bend** – 5 breaths each side

3 **Seated Twist** – 5 breaths each side

4 **Down Dog** – Bicycle out legs for 1 minute then shift forwards to Plank

5 **Plank** – 1 minute then shift back to Down Dog

6 **Down Dog** – 5 breaths

7 **Dolphin** – 5 breaths then shift forward to Dolphin Plank

8 **Dolphin Plank** – 1 minute then shift back to Dolphin

9 **Dolphin** – 5 breaths then push up to Down Dog

10 **Down Dog** – 5 breaths

11 **Mountain** – 5 breaths

12 **Thrive Sequence** – 3 rounds

13 **Child's Pose** – 1 minute

14 **Boat** – 5 breaths

15 **Low Boat** – 5 breaths

16 **Shoulder Squeezing Pose** – explore for 2 minutes

17 **Crow** – explore for 2 minutes

18 **Baby Bridge** – 5 breaths

19 **Reclining Twist** – 5 breaths each side

20 **Knees to Chest Pose** – 1 minute. Circle knees

21 **Corpse Pose** – 5–10 minutes

22 **Meditation**

Day 5: Stress-Proofing Your Body, Mind and Life

The stresses of the world can be very loud. Don't listen to them. For if you do, you won't be able to hear your heart.

Many of us live fast-paced, high-pressure lives, juggling demanding jobs with family responsibilities. On top of this we put pressure on ourselves to go to the gym, lose weight, host dinner parties, organise social get-togethers and generally keep everyone else happy. But living with an overwhelmed schedule often means existing with an underwhelmed soul.

Stress is an evolutionary adaptation. It came in handy when we were living in caves and had to run away from sabre-toothed tigers, but, in modern life (where we get stressed over everything from social media to not finishing everything on our to-do list), stress can be detrimental to our health.

It is mainly a physical response. The body thinks it is under attack so releases adrenaline, cortisol, norepinephrine and other hormones that prepare the body for action and shut down other functions such as digestion, rational thinking and immunity. We have three responses to this: fight, flight or freeze. We fight by taking our feelings out on ourselves, those we love and the world around us. We flee by running from the situation instead of facing it. Or we freeze and feel trapped and powerless.

Stress can come from many sources: comparison, competition, judgement, uncertainty, expectation, doubt, over-commitment, regret, worry, blame, guilt or overthinking.

I've learnt that a lot of the stress I carried was because I was hiding myself. I was pretending. I smiled when I wanted to cry and said yes when I wanted to say no. I was hiding because I felt ashamed and insecure and not good enough. Then slowly I stopped hiding. I cried when I needed to, asked for help from those I knew would never judge me and let go of the shame I had been carrying for so long. And life became easier.

When we reveal ourselves and acknowledge that we are human and that it is OK to melt down, we see that things have a way of working out. We begin to find the calm in the chaos and have the confidence to set healthy boundaries because we recognise that our time and energy are precious.

Stress is often a wake-up call that shows us that something in our life isn't right. It might be a job that is destroying our self-confidence, a relationship that isn't nourishing us or a diet that is draining us. It is up to us to find the lessons in stressful situations and stop giving our energy to things that are sucking the life out of us. That way we can tap into a peaceful state of mind and make wholehearted decisions about the direction of our life.

We are innately capable of handling whatever life throws at us without having a panic attack and there are several science-backed strategies to help reduce our stress levels when we're feeling overwhelmed:

- Going for a 10-minute walk in nature to boost endorphins and reduce stress hormones.
- Spending time with a good friend. Our close relationships serve as a buffer against negative situations.
- Mindfully snacking on a healthy wholefood. Nothing is more stressful to the brain than lacking nourishment.
- Turning off our phone and computer to give our brain a break from overstimulation.
- Listening to classical music to slow our heart rate and release dopamine and other feel-good neurochemicals.

Heart-Centred Exploration

The fact that we live stressful lives is undeniable. But just because our lives can be stressful does not mean that we have to get stressed out. Even if it feels like we are stuck in the middle of a storm it doesn't mean we have to let the storm get in us. One way we can do this is by creating a stress-free zone – a place that is free from deadlines, chores and to-do lists where you can read, write, draw, cry, laugh and do anything that will help you feel peaceful and relaxed.

If you have a spare room, then create a sanctuary with beautiful furniture, comfy cushions and calming paintings, leaving enough space for a yoga mat. Or, if you don't have much space at home, then create a corner of calm with an incense burner and fresh flowers. It doesn't matter how big the space is or what it looks like, as long as it gives you a feeling of peace and calm the minute you are in it.

Once you have created your stress-free space, make a list of everything that causes you stress in your life. It can include anything from your family not doing the washing-up to difficulties with your boss. Ban these things from your stress-free space so you can keep it as your place of calm in an often chaotic world.

De-Stress Sequence

Yoga helps us respond to stress with a balance of inner fire and inner calm. Today's sequence involves a Qi Gong exercise known as Shaking the Tree, which is something animals do very naturally to release physical stress from their bodies. You can find the full instructions for Shaking the Tree in the Yoga Pose Library on page 167.

Remember to set your intention before beginning the sequence. This will bring meaning to your practice and help you focus.

De-Stress Meditation

Our breath is one of the most powerful ways to stress-proof our lives. Imagine stress is a storm and your breath is an anchor. It won't make the storm pass any quicker, but it will keep you grounded until it does. Today's meditation uses a breathing exercise known as humming bee breath which research has found reduces stress levels and anxiety.

Begin in a comfortable seated position and push your index fingers gently into your ears to block out any sound. Take a deep inhale through your nose and as you exhale release a continuous humming sound. Focus on the vibration of the sound moving from your throat to your head. Once you've exhaled fully, inhale normally and repeat the humming on each exhale for three to five minutes.

Day 5: De-Stress Sequence

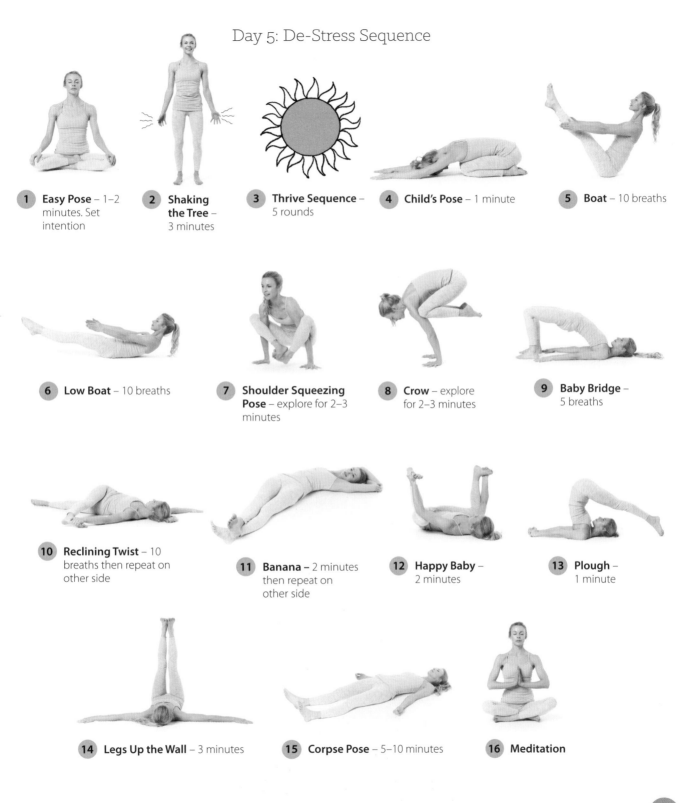

1 **Easy Pose** – 1–2 minutes. Set intention

2 **Shaking the Tree** – 3 minutes

3 **Thrive Sequence** – 5 rounds

4 **Child's Pose** – 1 minute

5 **Boat** – 10 breaths

6 **Low Boat** – 10 breaths

7 **Shoulder Squeezing Pose** – explore for 2–3 minutes

8 **Crow** – explore for 2–3 minutes

9 **Baby Bridge** – 5 breaths

10 **Reclining Twist** – 10 breaths then repeat on other side

11 **Banana** – 2 minutes then repeat on other side

12 **Happy Baby** – 2 minutes

13 **Plough** – 1 minute

14 **Legs Up the Wall** – 3 minutes

15 **Corpse Pose** – 5–10 minutes

16 **Meditation**

Day 6: Building Self-Compassion

You've let self-doubt and self-criticism run your life for years and it hasn't helped you heal. Try self-love and self-compassion and see what happens.

Life will throw whatever it wants at us. It will scatter us with kindness, love and happiness but it will also smack us with pain, stress and fear. Self-compassion allows us to relax and move towards our struggles so we reverse the self-critical messages we've been telling ourselves all our life. It creates a caring space within us that enables us to see our mistakes and insecurities with kindness and gentleness. It provides a powerful motivating force to help us reach our goals and chase our dreams because we are no longer fighting ourselves along the way.

We naturally feel compassion for those we love. If they are hurting, we want to relieve their pain. If they are upset, we want to comfort them. If they are lacking in confidence or doubting their place in the world, we treat them with gentleness and kindness, and reassure them that they are deserving of love and happiness.

But instead of treating ourselves with self-compassion when we are suffering or notice something about ourselves we don't like, we often turn to self-criticism, self-pity or self-indulgence.

Most us of believe that self-criticism is what keeps us motivated and, since we were children, we've learnt that being hard on ourselves is the way to be. When I was 12 years old I remember beating myself up when I got a B in a history essay, because I thought the more I criticised myself, the more motivated I would be to work harder for an A next time. The trouble is, self-criticism never gets us any closer to our goals. We can't shame ourselves into action.

Self-pity also comes naturally, but the problem with it is that we end up becoming immersed in our own struggles and get carried away in our emotional drama, leaving us feeling that we are alone. When we treat ourselves with self-compassion, this isolation and disconnection dissipates and we begin to understand that other people are suffering too. Our work stresses, relationship issues and worries about the size of our thighs become our link to humanity.

Self-indulgence is another way we cope with struggles instead of treating ourselves with self-compassion. Whether our stress leads to a splurge on designer handbags, a drunken night out, or an ice cream binge, these short-term pleasures may harm our long-term wellbeing. Self-compassion is about giving ourselves lasting health and happiness.

The Western world is obsessed with increasing self-esteem. And, while low self-esteem can lead to depression and anxiety, trying to increase it can be problematic because it often encourages us to ignore our imperfections instead of having compassion for these unwanted parts of ourselves. Unlike increasing self-esteem, which can take us on an emotional rollercoaster of superiority when we feel above average and insecurity when we don't meet our own high standards, increasing self-compassion empowers us to feel good about ourselves regardless of how pretty, smart, or popular we are, because we're human beings naturally worthy of respect.

Self-compassion can be anything from cooking ourselves a nourishing meal to making amends with the friend who we feel wronged us, because we don't want to carry the hurt with us any more. It includes:

- Treating ourselves with the same kindness we give to others.
- Accepting, forgiving, loving, respecting and protecting ourselves.
- Helping ourselves overcome our insecurities.
- Recognising painful emotions as they arise.
- Being gentle with ourselves when our self-esteem is low.
- Being aware of our own distress and being willing to help ourselves alleviate it.

Heart-Centred Exploration

Self-compassion requires three things: Being kind towards ourselves, feeling connected to others and being mindful. Today's exploration taps into these by asking you to acknowledge anything in your life that makes you feel like you are not good enough. Then, instead of judging yourself for these insecurities, treat yourself with love and kindness so you can overcome them.

Begin by making a list of all the things that make you feel inadequate. Notice what emotions you feel as you are doing this and, instead of suppressing them, allow yourself to feel them. Once you have made your list, imagine that you are an unconditionally loving and compassionate friend of yours.

Now write a letter to yourself from this friend. Focus on what they would say about your perceived failures and flaws, and how they would show compassion, acceptance and forgiveness by putting your health and happiness first. Be aware of how they reassure you that you do not need to earn happiness and love by being perfect or pleasing everyone – you deserve it for the simple reason that you are human. Keep this letter somewhere safe and return to it any time you feel your self-esteem has been knocked or you are in need of comfort and connection.

Self-Compassion Sequence

The yama, 'ahimsa' cultivates compassion. It translates as 'non-harm' so today's sequence focuses on being gentle with ourselves. The heart chakra is also closely related to compassion and any blockages can leave us feeling angry and self-loathing, so we'll also use backbends to release tension from the chest and open the heart.

Compassion Meditation

In today's meditation we will focus on compassion. Regularly practising self-compassion means that, regardless of whether we feel on top of the world, or we struggle to drag ourselves out of bed in the morning because we feel riddled with anxiety, we can recognise emotions rather than suppress them, and be gentle and kind to ourselves.

Begin by making a list of all the people you feel compassion towards – the people who, if they were suffering, you would want to be there for. Then begin to connect with that genuine compassion and experience what it feels like. Next, extend this compassion to yourself by creating an aspiration that works for you such as, *'May I be free from anxiety, stress and fear'.*

Close your eyes and begin to say this aspiration to yourself and connect with genuine compassion for yourself. If any feelings of guilt or shame arise, or any memories of failure pop into your mind, stay with the emotional distress rather than resist it and forgive yourself for being human. Once you have focused on self-compassion for a couple of minutes widen the circle of compassion to:

- Someone you love
- A friend
- A stranger or someone neutral
- Someone you find difficult or offensive
- All of the above equally
- All beings

Spend one to two minutes awakening compassion for each of the individuals and groups.

Day 6: Self-Compassion Sequence

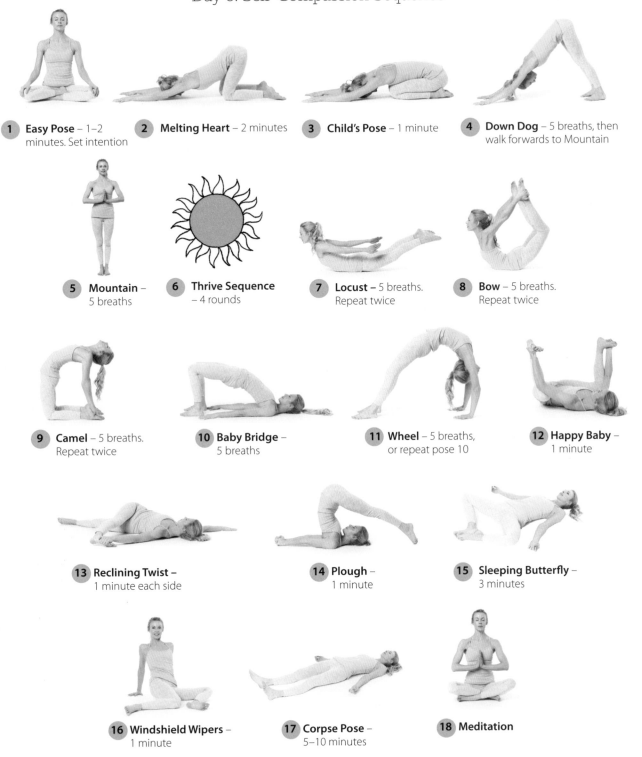

1 **Easy Pose** – 1–2 minutes. Set intention

2 **Melting Heart** – 2 minutes

3 **Child's Pose** – 1 minute

4 **Down Dog** – 5 breaths, then walk forwards to Mountain

5 **Mountain** – 5 breaths

6 **Thrive Sequence** – 4 rounds

7 **Locust** – 5 breaths. Repeat twice

8 **Bow** – 5 breaths. Repeat twice

9 **Camel** – 5 breaths. Repeat twice

10 **Baby Bridge** – 5 breaths

11 **Wheel** – 5 breaths, or repeat pose 10

12 **Happy Baby** – 1 minute

13 **Reclining Twist** – 1 minute each side

14 **Plough** – 1 minute

15 **Sleeping Butterfly** – 3 minutes

16 **Windshield Wipers** – 1 minute

17 **Corpse Pose** – 5–10 minutes

18 **Meditation**

Day 7: Overcoming Perfectionism

Your body. Your diet. Your life. It isn't perfect. It never was. It never will be. But it's real. It's honest. It's beautifully flawed. And totally magical.

The trouble with perfectionists is that most of us don't even realise we are one – we probably don't think we're perfect enough. Despite this, we carry around this idea that when our body, our work and our life is perfect, we will be worthy, loveable and happy. In reality, this constant striving for perfection doesn't protect us or motivate us, it keeps us trapped.

We live in a society where perfection is the goal – in school exams, in our career, in the cleanliness of our home, our diet, our parenting and relationships. Even the most beautiful of bodies are airbrushed to remove any slight imperfections. The more we can live up to these ideals of perfection, the worthier we believe we are as people. But if we ever do meet our own perfectionistic standards we quickly move our focus to another area of our life that we see as imperfect. We become trapped in a cycle of exhausting ourselves to meet our unrealistic expectations, while never feeling good enough.

The truth is, none of us are perfect. And that's OK. When we give up being perfect, we can start working on becoming a happier, kinder and more wholehearted version of ourselves. This means embracing that we have imperfections – because everybody does. It means embracing that our body is not perfect – because nobody's is. It means embracing that we are worth loving even though we have made mistakes and have flaws – because everyone has.

If you take a moment to think about someone you love: a partner, a parent or a child, you will begin to understand that you don't love them despite their imperfections, you love them with their imperfections, or even because of them. This is how we need to begin to see our own flaws. Once you've accepted your imperfections no one can use them against you. Not even you.

It has taken me a long time to embrace my imperfections – the things I used to beat myself up over: the bags under my eyes, the stretchmarks on my thighs, the way I speak too quickly when I meet new people, the multiple times I get my right and left mixed up when teaching a yoga class, the typos that miss the final edit, and the way I get oversensitive when I'm tired or hungry. But I have learnt that I will never be perfect. I can only be good enough.

We can waste our life hating our imperfections or we can accept them with compassion. Both routes can be challenging, but, with acceptance we will be happy one day, whereas with hatred we never will. Overcoming perfectionism involves:

- Believing we are good enough.
- Accepting our flaws.
- Setting realistic standards for ourselves and others.
- Being prepared to experiment, take risks and make mistakes.
- Putting more of ourselves into the world rather than hiding because we think we're not good enough.

Heart-Centred Exploration

The worse we feel about ourselves, the more we feel the need to be perfect. So, today's exploration looks at the infinite number of things we can aspire to be instead of chasing perfection. Pick at least 10 qualities from the following list that you aspire to be today and repeat the list to yourself as an aspiration as many times as you need to.

'May I be…	compassionate	fascinating	joyful	playful
accepting	confident	fearless	kind	present
adaptable	courageous	gentle	knowledgeable	relaxed
adventurous	creative	genuine	loving	strong
altruistic	daring	gracious	mindful	successful
ambitious	dependable	grateful	motivated	thoughtful
athletic	deserving	happy	nurturing	tranquil
authentic	desirable	healthy	open-hearted	understanding
beautiful	dynamic	hopeful	open-minded	unshakeable
brave	empowered	insightful	optimistic	vibrant
capable	energised	inspiring	passionate	wholehearted
caring	evolving	intuitive	peaceful	worthy

Self-Acceptance Sequence

Self-acceptance is the opposite of perfectionism. It is about recognising you are good enough just as you are. Today's sequence has some more challenging poses in it so instead of focusing on what the poses look like, focus on what they feel like. And remember, there is nothing to accomplish in yoga and no poses to perfect – just everything to endlessly explore.

Overcoming Perfectionism Meditation

It is our ego that drives our desire to be perfect so today's meditation focuses on releasing the ego and instead living from our heart, our consciousness, our true self – the spark that makes us *us*. This is known as 'So'hum' meditation and has been used for thousands of years because it is part of our nature – 'so' mimics the sounds of our inhalation, and 'hum' mimics the sound of our exhalation. The syllable 'so' means our consciousness and 'hum' means our ego. So, as we meditate, we are inhaling our consciousness and releasing our ego.

Begin in a comfortable seated position and take a couple of long, deep breaths. Silently begin to pronounce 'sooooo' on the inhalation and 'hummmm' on the exhalation. Repeat this mantra for 5–10 minutes, feeling the vibration release any desire for perfection and create a feeling of calm and groundedness.

Day 7: Self-Acceptance Sequence

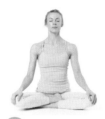 **1** **Easy Pose** – 1–2 minutes. Set intention

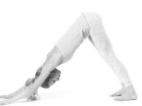 **2** **Down Dog** – 5 breaths, then walk forwards to Mountain

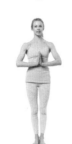 **3** **Mountain** – 5 breaths

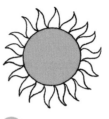 **4** **Thrive Sequence** – 4 rounds

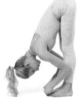 **5** **Standing Forward Bend** – 5 breaths

6 **Wide Legged Forward Bend** – 5 breaths

7 **Head to Knee Pose** – 5 breaths on each side

8 **Seated Forward Bend** – 5 breaths

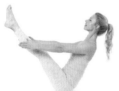 **9** **Boat** – 5 breaths. Repeat 3 times

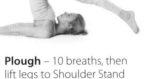 **10** **Plough** – 10 breaths, then lift legs to Shoulder Stand

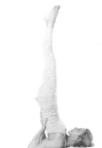 **11** **Shoulder Stand** – 10 breaths. Aim to get your body in a vertical line

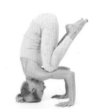 **12** **Egg Stand** – 10 breaths

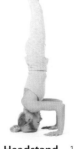 **13** **Headstand** – 10 breaths. Or stay in Egg Stand

14 **Caterpillar** – 1 minute

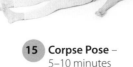 **15** **Corpse Pose** – 5–10 minutes

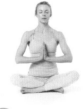 **16** **Meditation**

Day 8: Cultivating Gratitude

A grateful heart will transform your life.

Gratitude changes everything. It is nearly impossible to feel grateful and anxious at the same time so cultivating gratitude is one of the simplest and most powerful ways we can interrupt anxiety, stop stress, and awaken from depression.

As a society, we are addicted to talking about our problems. Whether it's that our job is too demanding, our partner isn't romantic enough or our belly is too wobbly, we find that complaining comes far more naturally than appreciating the fact that we have a job that pays well and allows us to spend time with our family, that our partner is always there when we need them, or that our belly was once home to our beautiful children. Gratitude shifts our focus from what our life lacks to the wonderful people, things, and experiences that are already present. And because gratitude doesn't always come naturally, it's important we take the time to cultivate it.

Gratitude has been a huge part of my own journey. I began keeping a gratitude diary when I was in recovery from anorexia and depression and wrote three things I was grateful for every day for over two years. On the days when it was painful to eat a bowl of cereal or even get out of bed I still found things to be grateful for: the view from my bedroom window, the love of my family, the promise of a new sunrise. And when I began a long-distance relationship, my partner and I would send each other gratitude texts every evening with three things we were grateful for so, although it hurt that we couldn't be together, we could share our appreciation of the things that made our lives beautiful.

When we refuse to become trapped by negative thoughts of guilt, entitlement and anxiety, and instead cultivate gratitude in our hearts, the world becomes a magical and amazing place – we unlock the fullness of life. Gratitude is a choice, and the more you live in a state of gratitude and constantly look for the good, the more present you become and the more you attract things to be grateful for.

Science has recognised the power of gratitude. Positive psychology research has found being grateful improves our physical health, increases self-esteem, energy and productivity, deepens relationships, helps us relax and enhances our overall wellbeing.

We can spend our life complaining about our current situation or we can choose to be grateful by:

- Appreciating all the positive things that come our way.
- Constantly looking for the good.
- Noticing the little things.
- Being aware of how much we have been given.
- Recognising the loving and supportive actions of others.
- Giving meaning to life by treating it as a gift.
- Living our life as if everything is a miracle.

Heart-Centred Exploration

When we're feeling anxious or stressed, those emotions and negative thoughts can override feeling grateful so we need to cultivate gratitude in our life by taking action. One of the simplest and most effective ways to do this is by creating a gratitude jar. The more we practise gratitude the stronger it gets, so this exploration is something we can do every day to retune our brain to look for the good in everything.

Simply get a large jar or box, place it by your bed or on your desk or anywhere you will see it regularly (you can decorate it if you like!) and place a notepad or some scrap paper beside it. At the end of each day, write down at least three things you are grateful for. It could be anything: something that made you smile, someone who has made your day more magical, something beautiful you notice about yourself, something new you've learned, a poem you've read or song you loved listening to. Fold up your gratitude note and pop it in the jar.

The gratitude jar serves two purposes: One, you strengthen your gratitude muscles by using them daily, and, two, in times of struggle, you can empty out the gratitude jar, read the notes, and be comforted by all the things you have to be grateful for.

Gratitude Sequence

The practice of gratitude brings balance to the heart chakra, and we can promote this balance through poses that focus on releasing tension from the chest and from around the heart.

Gratitude Meditation

One of the reasons we can struggle with feeling grateful is because we don't realise how many things in our life we take for granted – food, shelter, the people around us. This meditation helps you to cultivate gratitude for the simplest of things so that even when life is tough, we can still recognise how much we have in our life to appreciate.

Start off sitting comfortably and tune into your breath. Now, bring your awareness to your body, starting with your right foot and begin to imagine what your life would be like without it. How would you walk? How would you look? How would you feel if you no longer had your right foot? How would it restrict you or impact on your life? Now imagine what it would feel like getting it back; how you can run and dance and play sports, how easy life seems, and how much freedom you have.

Now bring your awareness to the room around you, your home. Imagine what life would be like without it. It might not be as big or as posh or as clean as you would like, but imagine not having it at all. Where would you sleep? Where would you cook? How would you feel being homeless? Now imagine getting your home back again. How does it feel to have shelter and warmth and comfort again?

Now recall what you had for breakfast and lunch today. Notice how it makes you feel. Satisfied? Fulfilled? Guilty? Imagine what it would be like not to have access to the foods that you enjoy or make you feel safe. How does it make you feel? Hungry? Scared? Weak? Now imagine getting those foods back again. How does it feel to have the foods you enjoy in your life again?

Now tune into your heart and visualise someone you love; a parent, child, partner, or friend. Imagine never speaking to them again. Feel the grief and the loss, the loneliness and heartbreak. Notice how you're no longer angry that they left dishes unwashed or they're always late or they have the TV on too loud – you just miss them. Now imagine them coming back into your life. Tune into the connection, love and joy you feel in your heart and allow that love to grow stronger in your daily life.

Take a few moments here to tune into what real gratitude feels like, and see if you can bring an element of it into your everyday life.

Day 8: Gratitude Sequence

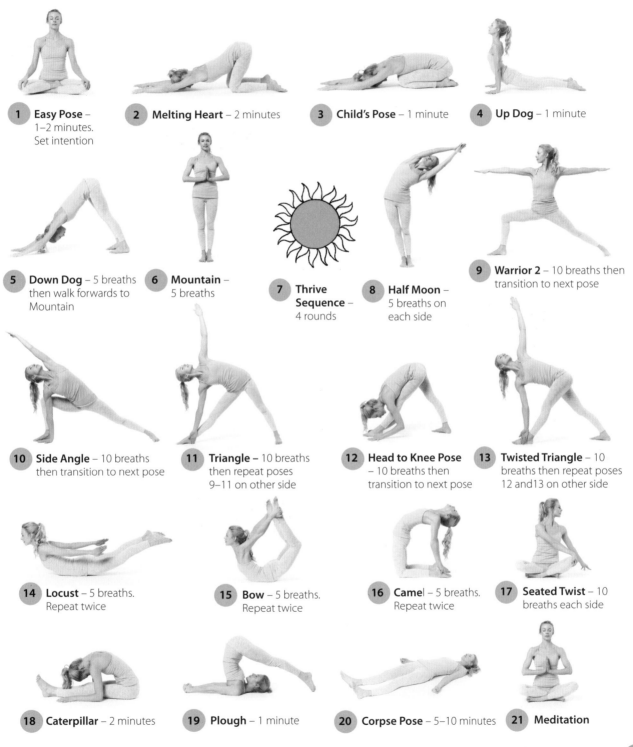

1 **Easy Pose** – 1–2 minutes. Set intention

2 **Melting Heart** – 2 minutes

3 **Child's Pose** – 1 minute

4 **Up Dog** – 1 minute

5 **Down Dog** – 5 breaths then walk forwards to Mountain

6 **Mountain** – 5 breaths

7 **Thrive Sequence** – 4 rounds

8 **Half Moon** – 5 breaths on each side

9 **Warrior 2** – 10 breaths then transition to next pose

10 **Side Angle** – 10 breaths then transition to next pose

11 **Triangle** – 10 breaths then repeat poses 9–11 on other side

12 **Head to Knee Pose** – 10 breaths then transition to next pose

13 **Twisted Triangle** – 10 breaths then repeat poses 12 and 13 on other side

14 **Locust** – 5 breaths. Repeat twice

15 **Bow** – 5 breaths. Repeat twice

16 **Camel** – 5 breaths. Repeat twice

17 **Seated Twist** – 10 breaths each side

18 **Caterpillar** – 2 minutes

19 **Plough** – 1 minute

20 **Corpse Pose** – 5–10 minutes

21 **Meditation**

Day 9: Facing Fear and Finding Freedom

Sometimes the things we fear the most are the very things that will set us free.

Fear of failure, fear of success, fear of what other people think, fear of being fat, fear of being ugly, fear of being lonely, fear of taking risks, fear of change, fear of staying the same… Most of us have fears that keep us trapped. This feeling of being restricted, caged and imprisoned by anxiety and worry is the opposite of freedom. And the key to thriving and finding freedom is to let go of fear. This doesn't necessarily mean we don't feel fear any more; it means that we handle fear in a way that softens us and allows us to move gently towards it so that whatever scares us no longer has power or restricts our lives.

We grow the most when we are outside of our comfort zone. But the truth is, anytime we venture outside of our comfort zone we are going to feel some fear. The usual coping strategies for fear are avoidance, hopelessness (where we lose insight into what will bring us relief), and resentment (where we condemn and criticise ourselves for our fear). I even thought that I could think my way out of fear – that the more I worried about whatever scared me, the more I could control it. I was wrong. While these strategies may bring us relief for a while, they are futile and will keep us trapped. At some point we will start to question, *'why am I scared?'* and, *'why do my fears keep growing bigger every year?'*

I've been trapped by those prisons of fear. And, looking back, I was trapped because I didn't know there was an alternative. I thought that I would fear food and my body forever. I thought that I would feel controlled and repressed in all relationships. I thought that stress and anxiety were just part and parcel of life. Now that I know there is an alternative I have consciously created a life of freedom – the freedom to eat, to work and to love as I choose. And I've learnt that, instead of resisting and avoiding my fears, I had to fully experience them and become inquisitive about them in order to find freedom.

Fear is a trigger for action. When we feel fear we need to do something, anything. Only when I understood this could I eat the foods that scared me, take the risk to leave the relationship that no longer nourished me, and be brave enough to walk away from the job that left me feeling unfulfilled.

Another big lesson I learnt on my own journey is that fear is a *choice*. It is a product of the thoughts we create and the stories we tell ourselves. Psychologists have found that we can reappraise fear and anxiety as excitement, because both anxiety and excitement are aroused emotions – our heart beats faster, our palms get sweaty and our level of cortisol surges as our body prepares for action. The only difference is that when we are fearful, we focus on all the things that can go wrong and when we are excited we focus on all the ways something could go well.

Feeling fear is a sign there is something important to overcome. Instead of ignoring it or avoiding it, we can gently move towards it, understand it, and feel excited about the freedom we will experience when we discover that we can do what we were afraid we couldn't do.

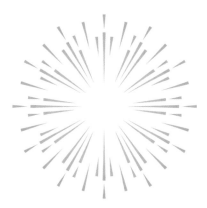

Heart-Centred Exploration

Fear is the opposite of feeling stable and secure so signifies an imbalance in our root chakra. A simple way to bring this chakra back into balance and to help us feel more grounded is through a process called 'earthing'. All this means is walking barefoot on the earth, or laying in the grass so your physical body is in direct contact with the ground. Emerging scientific evidence shows that when we reconnect with the electrons on the earth's surface the electrons transfer to our body and promote wellbeing. This includes regulating our stress hormones, which can help us feel more grounded and less fearful so we can live with greater freedom. So today's exploration asks you to spend 5–10 minutes barefoot on the grass reconnecting to the earth. This is a lovely thing to do first thing in the morning as part of your daily routine.

Facing Fear Sequence

Fear of falling and fear of failing are two fears that most of us experience regularly. Today's yoga sequence includes some challenging poses that might induce fear and that you might fall out of. If you are scared about practising any of the poses, I encourage you to become inquisitive and understand why. Are you afraid of falling? Hurting yourself? Of not being able to do the pose perfectly? Once you've understood your fear, take action and explore the poses with compassion. And, if you do fall, enjoy it. Imperfection is freedom.

Facing Fear Meditation

The key to freedom is presence. Fear keeps us trapped in the past or worried about the future. When we recognise and move towards our fear we begin to realise that, right now, we are OK. Today's meditation uses a technique called 'noting' to identify our fears without becoming caught up in the stories that come with them. This allows us to relax into the emotional energy and sit with our fears so that they no longer have power over us.

Begin in a comfortable seated position and bring your awareness to your breath by focusing on the rise and fall of your belly. Now awaken the feeling of fear by thinking of something that scares you. It could be a common fear like spiders or snakes, or something more personal that holds you back like the fear of gaining weight, making a mistake at work or people not liking you. Focus on this fear for a moment or two and label it with a mental note like 'thinking', 'memory', 'fearing', or 'pain'. Avoid getting too sucked into the detail. For example, if you feel anxious about failing an exam, label it 'failing' or 'anxiety' instead of 'failing an exam'.

Return your awareness to your breath and if another source of fear or anxiety comes to mind, take a moment or two to label it and then bring your awareness back to your breath.

Spend 5–10 minutes doing this so that you begin to observe your fears without attaching to them. This will help us to see that it is our fear, rather than what we are afraid of, that is causing our unhappiness.

Day 9: Facing Fear Sequence

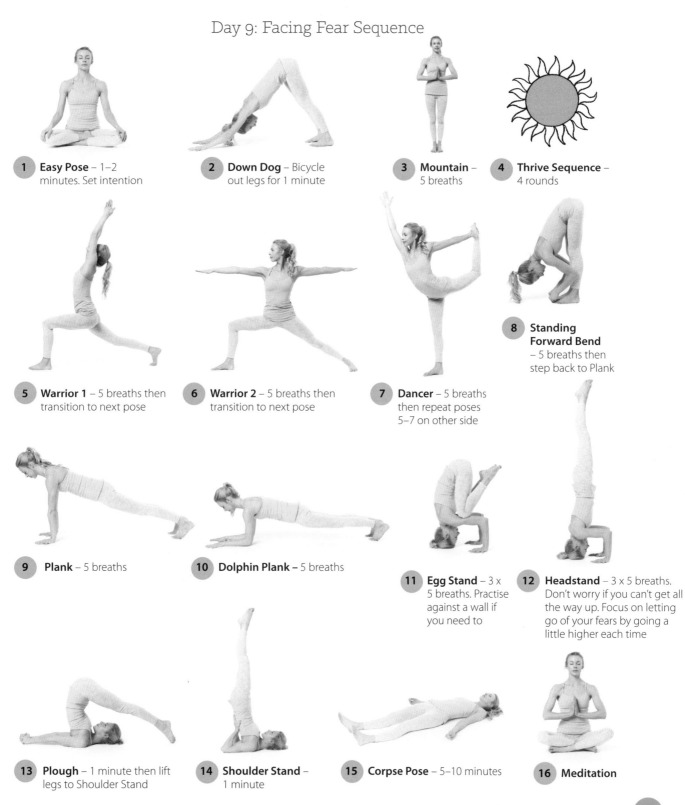

1 **Easy Pose** – 1–2 minutes. Set intention

2 **Down Dog** – Bicycle out legs for 1 minute

3 **Mountain** – 5 breaths

4 **Thrive Sequence** – 4 rounds

5 **Warrior 1** – 5 breaths then transition to next pose

6 **Warrior 2** – 5 breaths then transition to next pose

7 **Dancer** – 5 breaths then repeat poses 5–7 on other side

8 **Standing Forward Bend** – 5 breaths then step back to Plank

9 **Plank** – 5 breaths

10 **Dolphin Plank** – 5 breaths

11 **Egg Stand** – 3 x 5 breaths. Practise against a wall if you need to

12 **Headstand** – 3 x 5 breaths. Don't worry if you can't get all the way up. Focus on letting go of your fears by going a little higher each time

13 **Plough** – 1 minute then lift legs to Shoulder Stand

14 **Shoulder Stand** – 1 minute

15 **Corpse Pose** – 5–10 minutes

16 **Meditation**

Day 10: Igniting Your Inner Fire

*Don't let anyone stop you from doing the things
that set your soul on fire. Not even you.*

When we are stressed, anxious or afraid, it's easy to let our inner fire go out. It's easy to get so caught up in the worries and demands of daily life that we lose sight of our passions and resign ourselves to a life that doesn't fulfil us. The truth is, the life you dream of does exist. It is real. It is possible. And you do deserve it.

As kids our inner fire burned brightly. We climbed trees, did cartwheels and jumped in streams because we were excited for life. But at some point we stopped doing what we loved and started doing what was expected of us.

Fire symbolises passion and creation. It is our energy, courage and hunger for life. There are times when we all feel like our fire has gone out. But, just like a phoenix which rises from the ashes, we can reawaken our passions and live a more meaningful and fulfilling life.

When I was struggling with anorexia, anxiety and depression, it felt as if I was lost in the fire. I no longer had passions, I had obsessions. I had stopped doing all the things I loved because I was so consumed by calorie counting and compulsions. My inner fire had gone out. Then I stumbled across yoga and it started a fire within me that could not die. Instead of feeling lost in the fire, I felt as though I could rebuild myself from it. Yoga sparked a journey of self-discovery that burned away all the things that were holding me back. And, from that little spark, my passion for life was reignited and I began to heal.

It was yoga that reawakened my passion for life, but it could be anything or anyone. If our fire has been out for some time then it can take a little while to reignite and we may have to explore new hobbies and pastimes, surround ourselves with new people and spend time in different places. But it will always reignite while doing something that excites us and makes us feel alive.

We may already know what our passion is – the thing that makes our heart beat faster and eyes shine brighter when we do it or think about it, but we are too afraid to follow it because we have a stable job, a mortgage to pay and we think we're too old. We resign ourselves to a practical life instead of a passionate one because there is a certain amount of bravery needed to acknowledge and embrace our passions. However, creating as many passionate moments as possible is what life is all about. And when we do, it will allow us to heal, grow and thrive.

According to Ayurveda, having a strong inner fire (known as *'agni'*), is crucial to our health and wellbeing. It is what helps us weather the storm when life gets tough. To keep it burning brightly we need to live life more consciously, minimise things that deplete our energy and be brave enough to fully devote ourselves to following our heart. Only then will we have the drive, enthusiasm and limitless energy to face our fears, own our worth and be the best versions of ourselves we can be.

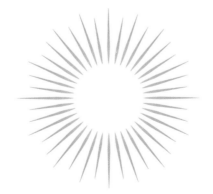

Heart-Centred Exploration

Igniting our inner fire can take time, especially when we're going through a period of stress and anxiety. We don't need to worry about finding our life purpose or try to change the world at this stage. Instead, by focusing on small things that excite us each day, we will discover our passion, and over time, this will connect us to our purpose in life.

Today's exploration is about reigniting our childhood passions. Find a quiet space and begin by writing down the things you used to enjoy doing from the ages of 5 to 15. What hobbies did you have? What after-school clubs were you a member of? What books did you enjoy reading? What did you do at weekends? Often, we'll remember that it's the simple things that gave us the most joy – making cupcakes with our grandma, picnics at the beach, our parents reading us bedtime stories, or having egg and spoon races.

Once you have a list of your childhood passions see how you can integrate them into your adult life. Bake a cake, go for a wander along the seafront, read a new book or sign up to an obstacle race and start training. Whatever you do, do it for its own sake. Don't worry about what your cake looks like or how fast you can complete the obstacle race. When we feel excited about doing activities with no ulterior motive other than enjoyment, we recreate the childlike state of pure passion and reignite our love for life.

Inner Fire Sequence

Traditionally, in Ayurveda and yoga, our inner fire is said to reside in our belly – our solar plexus chakra. Today's sequence focuses on strengthening our inner fire using core-based poses and arm balances.

Inner Fire Meditation

The inner fire meditation uses the mantra 'RAM' to strengthen the power of our solar plexus chakra and burn away any limiting beliefs that no longer serve us so our energy can flow freely. Mantras are simple words or phrases that create soundwave energy to promote healing and personal growth. The vibrations are said to stimulate certain parts of the brain to leave you feeling relaxed and revitalised.

Begin in a comfortable seated position and take a couple of long deep breaths. Place your right hand over your belly so your palm is resting just below your belly button, and place your left palm on top of your right. Visualise the area beneath your palm filling with a golden light. Take a deep breath in and as you exhale say 'RAAAAAAAAAAAAAAAM'. Repeat for a couple of minutes, taking deep inhalations and repeating the mantra 'RAAAAAAAAAAAAAAAM' as you breathe out. Feel the vibration of the sound and notice the heat and energy flowing through your solar plexus chakra as you awaken the fire within.

Day 10: Inner Fire Sequence

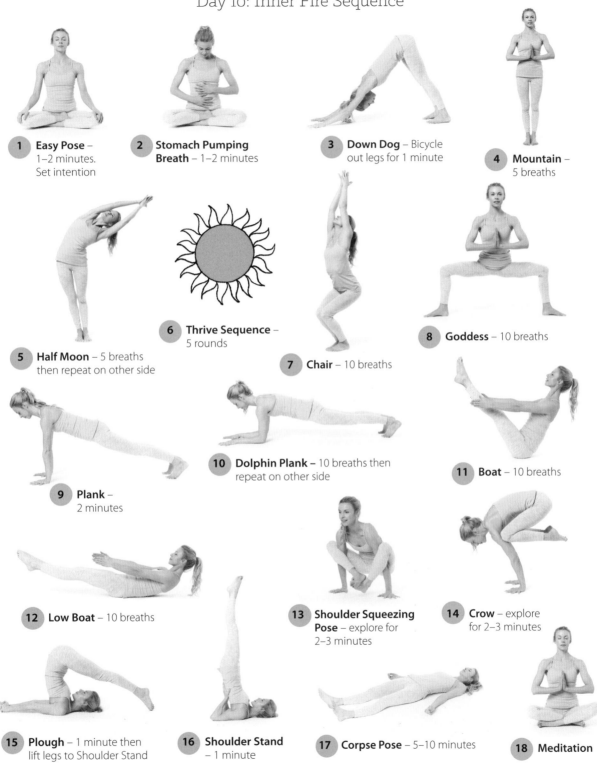

1 **Easy Pose** – 1–2 minutes. Set intention

2 **Stomach Pumping Breath** – 1–2 minutes

3 **Down Dog** – Bicycle out legs for 1 minute

4 **Mountain** – 5 breaths

5 **Half Moon** – 5 breaths then repeat on other side

6 **Thrive Sequence** – 5 rounds

7 **Chair** – 10 breaths

8 **Goddess** – 10 breaths

9 **Plank** – 2 minutes

10 **Dolphin Plank** – 10 breaths then repeat on other side

11 **Boat** – 10 breaths

12 **Low Boat** – 10 breaths

13 **Shoulder Squeezing Pose** – explore for 2–3 minutes

14 **Crow** – explore for 2–3 minutes

15 **Plough** – 1 minute then lift legs to Shoulder Stand

16 **Shoulder Stand** – 1 minute

17 **Corpse Pose** – 5–10 minutes

18 **Meditation**

Day 11: Discovering Your True Strength

When life puts us to the test we all have an unexpected reserve of strength inside of us that allows us to grow in ways we never imagined we could.

Life can be tough. Every day we're faced with challenges at home, at work and in our relationships. Some days life will knock us completely off balance leaving us questioning whether we'll ever feel strong again. We can't always change these situations – the relationship breakups, the redundancies, or the loss of loved ones. But by discovering our true strength we can wait for these storms to pass patiently and courageously instead of being struck down by them.

A greater sense of personal strength is one of the elements that has been found in research on post-traumatic growth. When we are faced with some kind of struggle in our lives, we can treat it as an opportunity to transform ourselves and see the world with a fresh outlook. For example, if we are going through a period of depression, stress or anxiety, instead of resisting it or wallowing in it, it can introduce new strengths that we wouldn't have known existed within us. We don't need to let worry control us, or stress break us.

I've been there too. I spent years completely oblivious to my true strength. I felt like a victim and was desperate for someone to pull me out of my crisis and make me feel normal again. Then I realised that the only person who could do that was me. It was me who had the strength to nourish my body with good food. It was me who had the strength to let go of the worries and the anxieties. It was me who had the strength to rebuild my whole life. And it is incredibly empowering to know that we have the strength to do this – to transform ourselves.

It takes true strength to let go of what no longer nourishes us, face our fears, and work through every other chapter in this book. This is why the heart-centred explorations, yoga sequences and meditations are so important. They help us to:

1. **Reflect on what we have overcome before**
   We often underestimate our true strength. One of the best ways to see how strong we really are is to look back on the times where we have survived storms we never thought we could. This will also help us to see above our current struggles and remind us that we are bigger and stronger than whatever is going on in our lives right now.

2. **Be motivated by outer strength**
   True strength is about more than how much weight we can lift or how long we can hold a handstand, but in order to feel strong holistically we have to build a foundation of physical strength. There is no separation between our body and our mind, so as we build physical strength through our yoga practice we also cultivate strength within.

3. **Develop and nurture a spiritual connection**
   Spiritual change is another one of the elements of thriving found in research. Spirituality involves having a sense of connection to something bigger than ourselves so we feel that we are part of something greater. This reduces feelings of alienation and isolation, and allows us to accept guidance and comfort from other human beings, the universe, or whatever higher power we believe in so that we access a source of strength and resilience within us.

Heart-Centred Exploration

One of the first steps to developing true strength is to identify and embrace our natural strengths. We are all good at different things – some of us run fast, others are great at physics and some of us can paint beautiful artwork.

Two psychology researchers, Professor Chris Peterson and Dr. Martin Seligmen, have identified 24 character strengths grouped under six categories so, for today's exploration, use the following list of strengths and identify how you have demonstrated this strength in the past, or how you can use it in the future. This will put whatever struggle you are going through into perspective so that it's not so overwhelming and you can understand that you have the strength to deal with it.

Character strengths

- Wisdom: What are you curious about in life? What do you love learning? What advice do you offer friends when they come to you for help?

- Courage: How do you express bravery (e.g. speaking up for what you believe in)? What goals are you working towards despite obstacles and challenges? How are you honest with yourself about your feelings, goals, and relationships?

- Humanity: How do you express love to your parents or children? Your partner? A friend? Yourself? What random acts of kindness do you perform? How are you friendly?

- Justice: What's your role in a team? How do you express fairness (e.g. by treating others the way you would like to be treated)? Who is your favourite leader and how do they inspire you?

- Temperance: How do you show forgiveness? When friends come to you and share their achievements and accomplishments how to do you react? Do you allow them the limelight? In what ways do you think before you act?

- Transcendence: How do you show appreciation for the beautiful things in the world (e.g. art, nature, books)? How do you express gratitude? How do you stay positive and optimistic? What makes you laugh? How do you bring an element of the sacred into your everyday life?

. . . .

True Strength Sequence

Physical strength and inner strength cannot be separated. As our body gets stronger through exercise and yoga, our mind becomes more resilient in overcoming challenges. Lots of research has shown that exercise, especially yoga, is an effective way to treat depression and anxiety, so today's sequence focuses on building physical and mental strength through dynamic flows and challenging balances.

. . . .

True Strength Meditation

In today's meditation, we use an aspiration to build strength so that even if we don't feel strong enough to take action, we can still aspire to.

Begin by finding a comfortable seated position and close your eyes. Start by developing a feeling of personal strength by reflecting on the strengths you discovered in today's heart centred exploration. Embrace this strength in an aspiration such as: *'May I be strong enough to use my struggles and my joys as vehicles for transformation.'*

Once you cultivate this feeling of personal strength, see if you can widen the circle of strength to someone you love by using an aspiration such as: *'May my mum be strong enough to use her struggles and her joys as vehicles for transformation.'* Once you have awakened this feeling of strength for someone you love, do the same for:

- A friend
- A stranger or someone neutral
- Someone you find difficult or offensive
- All of the above equally
- All beings

Spend one to two minutes awakening strength for each of the individuals and groups.

Day 11: True Strength Sequence

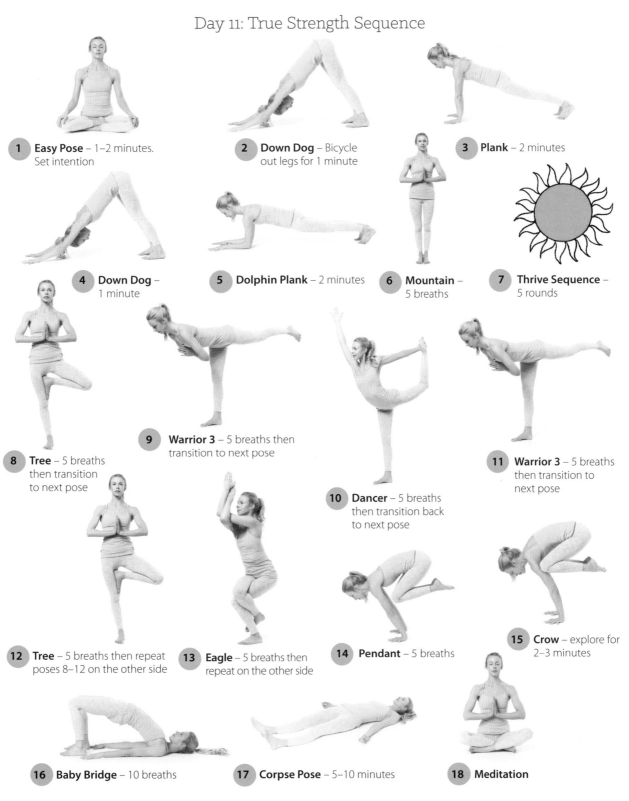

1 **Easy Pose** – 1–2 minutes. Set intention

2 **Down Dog** – Bicycle out legs for 1 minute

3 **Plank** – 2 minutes

4 **Down Dog** – 1 minute

5 **Dolphin Plank** – 2 minutes

6 **Mountain** – 5 breaths

7 **Thrive Sequence** – 5 rounds

8 **Tree** – 5 breaths then transition to next pose

9 **Warrior 3** – 5 breaths then transition to next pose

10 **Dancer** – 5 breaths then transition back to next pose

11 **Warrior 3** – 5 breaths then transition to next pose

12 **Tree** – 5 breaths then repeat poses 8–12 on the other side

13 **Eagle** – 5 breaths then repeat on the other side

14 **Pendant** – 5 breaths

15 **Crow** – explore for 2–3 minutes

16 **Baby Bridge** – 10 breaths

17 **Corpse Pose** – 5–10 minutes

18 **Meditation**

Day 12: Loving Your Body

When you stop worrying about having a beautiful body, you can start building a beautiful life. And this life will bring you more happiness than a flat stomach and a perfect butt ever could.

Nobody ever tells us that it's OK to call ourselves beautiful. Nobody ever says that we can love our waist and our hips and our thighs. Nobody ever says its OK to compliment our assets instead of moaning about our flaws. So I'll say it now:

You are allowed to love your body exactly the way it is.

There is no wonder that over 60 per cent of us are ashamed of our bodies with the rise of selfies on social media becoming a breeding ground for judgement and comparison, and magazines boasting front covers telling us how to get *'slim and sexy'*, *'lose inches all over'* and *'be bulge-free'*. The problem with these messages is that not only do we feel we need to lose inches, we also lose self-confidence, self-compassion and self-love.

Media isn't the only problem when it comes to loving our body. We can be our own worst enemy. We think that degrading our body is a form of modesty when actually it just weakens our spirit. We think that if we criticise our body enough it will lead to change when in reality the criticism just keeps us trapped in a cycle of binging or starving or whatever destructive coping mechanisms we've become caught up in. The truth is, we can't hate our body into loving it. And in reality, our body was never the problem in the first place. There is nothing wrong with its scars, stretch marks, lumps and bumps. Our curves, wrinkles, smooth places and wobbly bits are just fine as they are. Do we really want to spend our one precious life hating our thighs, condemning our bellies, and wishing we were thinner, curvier, taller, shorter, with a smaller nose, bigger boobs and longer legs?

It took me a long time to love my body, to learn that my worth does not depend on how much I weigh or how flat my stomach is, and to realise that the way my belly has softened and thigh gap has shrunk does not make me any less beautiful. Since my journey through anorexia 10 years ago, my body has changed a lot. My thighs are bigger, my belly is softer, my face is rounder. My heart is healthier, my bones are stronger and my skin is brighter. But the thing that has changed more than my body is my mind. I've realised the things that I thought were important – weight, calories, the circumference of my waist, wearing a size 4 … are not so important after all. I've learnt that our body is precious. It is our vehicle for thriving and we need to take good care of it.

When we stop criticising ourselves in the mirror we can turn our gaze inwards and focus on the things that really matter – our dreams, our relationships, our personal growth. Instead of worrying about how big our bum looks, we can use our energy to be comfortable with ourselves and figure out what we have to share with the world.

Many of us spend our lives fighting to change our body to fit some kind of ideal. But research shows those of us who fit that ideal are just as likely to be unhappy with our bodies as those who don't. So the other option is to change our attitude towards our body – to appreciate it instead of criticise it, to nourish it instead of punish it and to love it instead of hate it. Developing this body confidence means we:

- Accept ourselves as we are.

- Realise that our body isn't perfect, *but no one else's is either.*

- Don't feel the need to change our weight or have plastic surgery to feel better about ourselves.

- May still want to improve our body by losing or gaining weight or toning up but know it won't make us any more valuable as a person.

Heart-Centred Exploration

Even if we admit to hating our body, there will be times when we transcend this self-criticism and feel in love with ourselves and with life. So, for today's exploration, document the moments you feel most in love with yourself. What were you doing? Who were you with? Where were you? What were you wearing? How were you feeling?

Once you've made a list of these moments, see if you can identify a common theme. Maybe you feel most in love with your body when you're around a specific friend or partner. Or it might be when you're in nature or when you're playing sport. See if you can recreate these body positive experiences as often as you can.

Body Love Sequence

When we love our body, regardless of what we would like to change about it, we create a mind-set of self-respect and body appreciation that means we make healthy lifestyle choices that will nourish us. Today's sequence focuses on our heart chakra. It includes heart-opening poses that will allow love for our body to flow freely, as well as hip openers that will shift our focus from what our body looks like to how it feels.

Body Love Meditation

Deep breaths are like little love notes to your body. They send a simple message that you care about your health and your happiness. Today's meditation uses a pranayama (a traditional yogic breathing exercise) known as 'equal breathing'. By deepening each inhale and lengthening each exhale you slow down the nervous system, reduce anxiety and nourish your body with oxygen.

Begin seated and take a couple of long deep breaths into your belly. Once you've found your focus on your breath, begin inhaling for a count of four and exhaling for a count of four. Breathe through your nose, increasing the length to a count of six or eight if you can. Breathe like this for up to 10 minutes and then slowly allow your breathing rate to return to normal.

At times of stress or when you find yourself criticising your body, return to this equal breathing method to slow your mind down and remind yourself that you are worthy of nourishing with deep breaths, kind thoughts and self-love.

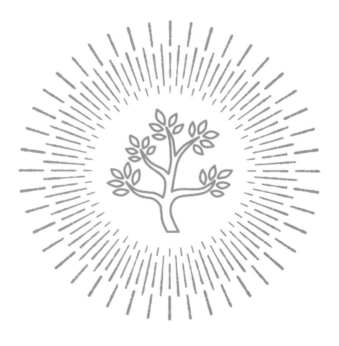

Day 12: Body Love Sequence

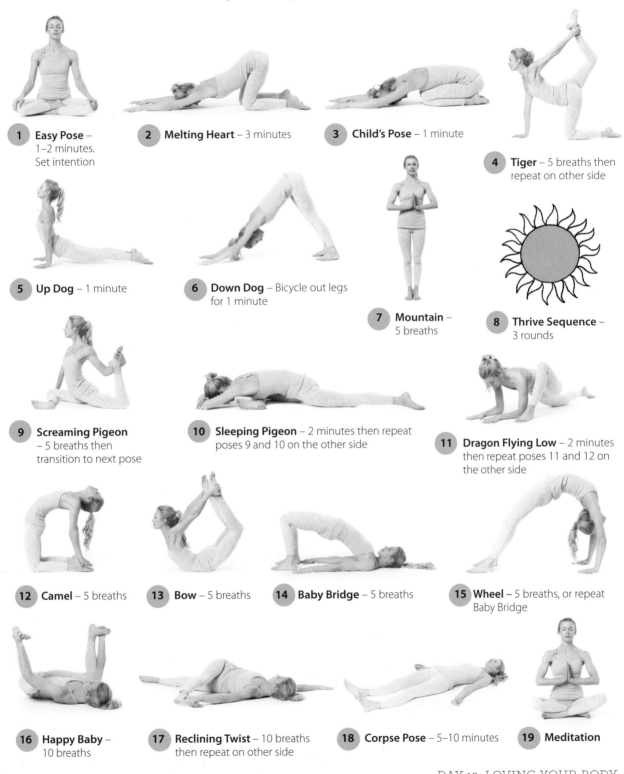

1 **Easy Pose** – 1–2 minutes. Set intention

2 **Melting Heart** – 3 minutes

3 **Child's Pose** – 1 minute

4 **Tiger** – 5 breaths then repeat on other side

5 **Up Dog** – 1 minute

6 **Down Dog** – Bicycle out legs for 1 minute

7 **Mountain** – 5 breaths

8 **Thrive Sequence** – 3 rounds

9 **Screaming Pigeon** – 5 breaths then transition to next pose

10 **Sleeping Pigeon** – 2 minutes then repeat poses 9 and 10 on the other side

11 **Dragon Flying Low** – 2 minutes then repeat poses 11 and 12 on the other side

12 **Camel** – 5 breaths

13 **Bow** – 5 breaths

14 **Baby Bridge** – 5 breaths

15 **Wheel** – 5 breaths, or repeat Baby Bridge

16 **Happy Baby** – 10 breaths

17 **Reclining Twist** – 10 breaths then repeat on other side

18 **Corpse Pose** – 5–10 minutes

19 **Meditation**

Day 13: Letting Your Emotions be in Motion

Never apologise for having too much emotion, for being too sensitive, or for feeling too deeply. These are your superpowers. Don't hide them from the world.

Emotions make us human. They make us real. We've got to feel them, express them, and move through them for us to be healthy.

In a society that values logic and rationale, many of us bottle up our painful emotions out of fear of being seen as too sensitive, needy or weak. We numb them out with work or food or alcohol because we want to avoid the pain. But when we fight against difficult emotions, we get trapped by them.

Repressed emotions block our energy and break down the mind, body and spirit. They exhaust us and make us sick. Several research studies have found a strong link between the suppression of toxic emotions like anger, hate and resentment, and the development of cancer and other chronic illnesses. When we repress painful emotions our stress hormones increase, which suppresses our immune system and can allow normal cells to mutate into cancer cells.

We are not robots. We are allowed to feel. We can't think our way out of pain or logic our way out of emotion. We have to feel it. This doesn't mean we need to analyse why we're feeling a negative emotion or justify why we don't feel good – this just wastes our energy and only adds more power to the pain.

Instead, we need to listen to our emotions and the messages they are giving us. For example, anger shows us what we're passionate about and what we believe needs changing in the world. Shame shows us that we are internalising other people's judgements and need to reconnect with ourselves. Anxiety shows us that we need to be present. Disappointment shows us that we still care about something or someone. Discomfort shows us that we've been given the opportunity to change and to grow.

It is our emotions that lead to action. When I was going through anorexia I made so many lists of the logical pros and cons of living with anorexia. The negatives always outweighed the positives. But it wasn't until I allowed myself to truly feel the powerlessness, shame, guilt, regret and despair that I took action and began to heal.

One of the reasons those of us who go through periods of stress, anxiety and depression so often numb our emotions is because we are highly sensitive. We feel everything intensely and sometimes it becomes overwhelming. Embracing our sensitivity instead of suppressing it may mean we suffer more but we also love harder, dream bigger, experience deeper connection and have a greater appreciation for the little things. Our sensitivity is our strength and, when we engage with and allow our emotions to be in motion, it is what makes us feel truly alive.

Emotions can be exhausting, which is why the need for self-care is essential. And just like we educate the mind, we can educate the heart so we can use the energy of our emotions effectively. This is known as emotional intelligence and includes:

- The ability to sense, understand and apply the power of emotions as a source of energy, connection and influence.
- Knowing our strengths, weaknesses, drives, values and goals and the impact they have on others.
- Feeling an emotion without having to act on it.
- Using gut feelings to guide decisions.
- Being empathic and suspending our egos so we can live in another's world.

Heart-Centred Exploration

One of the reasons we suppress our emotions is because we don't know how to identify or express them – it feels like we just don't have the words. For today's exploration make a list of emotion words (both positive and negative) such as those below. Once you have made a list, experiment with working these words into your vocabulary so you can identify and express emotions you would usually avoid.

Acceptance	Excitement	Hate	Love	Shame
Anger	Fear	Hope	Overwhelm	Sorrow
Boredom	Frustration	Impatience	Peace	Trust
Courage	Grief	Insecurity	Powerlessness	Understanding
Disappointment	Guilt	Jealousy	Pride	Unworthiness
Enthusiasm	Happiness	Joy	Regret	Worry

Emotions in Motion Sequence

Emotion is energy in motion so today's sequence uses a flow of poses to release blockages and allow your energy to flow freely. By matching your movement with your breath you will bring your awareness to the present moment and give your emotions space to be felt and released.

Emotional Intelligence Meditation

Allowing our emotions to be in motion means feeling the feeling but not becoming the emotion. Witness it, allow it and then release it. Today's meditation is a visualisation inspired by words from the Buddhist teacher, Pema Chödrön:

'You are the sky. Everything else is just the weather.'

Begin in a comfortable seated position and allow your awareness to settle on your natural breathing rhythm. Now visualise the sky – crystal clear, bright blue, vast and endless. Imagine that this sky, full of brightness and beauty, is you.

Now allow anything you've been suppressing to come to mind – emotions, situations, challenges. Visualise these difficulties as clouds in the sky. They might be big angry looking grey clouds or small white fluffy ones.

Focus on one of these clouds at a time, and as you do, allow yourself to feel whatever arises without justifying it or getting caught up in the story line. Now visualise a gentle breeze blowing this cloud across the sky until it disappears. Do the same with all the other clouds in your sky – identify it, feel the energy of the emotion and then allow it to pass until all you are left with is a clear blue sky.

Day 13: Emotions in Motion Sequence

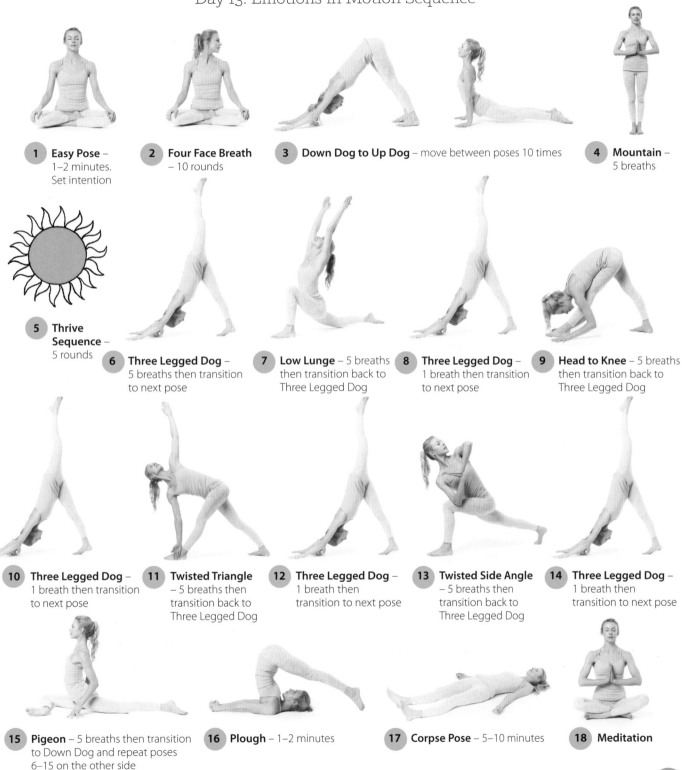

1 Easy Pose – 1–2 minutes. Set intention

2 Four Face Breath – 10 rounds

3 Down Dog to Up Dog – move between poses 10 times

4 Mountain – 5 breaths

5 Thrive Sequence – 5 rounds

6 Three Legged Dog – 5 breaths then transition to next pose

7 Low Lunge – 5 breaths then transition back to Three Legged Dog

8 Three Legged Dog – 1 breath then transition to next pose

9 Head to Knee – 5 breaths then transition back to Three Legged Dog

10 Three Legged Dog – 1 breath then transition to next pose

11 Twisted Triangle – 5 breaths then transition back to Three Legged Dog

12 Three Legged Dog – 1 breath then transition to next pose

13 Twisted Side Angle – 5 breaths then transition back to Three Legged Dog

14 Three Legged Dog – 1 breath then transition to next pose

15 Pigeon – 5 breaths then transition to Down Dog and repeat poses 6–15 on the other side

16 Plough – 1–2 minutes

17 Corpse Pose – 5–10 minutes

18 Meditation

Day 14: Finding Balance

Finding balance in a world of extremes is a skill very few have mastered. But when you learn to live in the magical space between effort and surrender you will discover that life flows more beautifully than ever.

If we want to thrive, finding balance is a necessity. Balance is the key to everything. When we find it, we feel good and look good, we are full of energy and vitality, and we become both perfectly peaceful and wonderfully wild.

Balance is about control and surrender. It's about knowing when to hold on and when to let go, when to drink smoothies and when to eat cake, when to party all night and when to stay in our pyjamas and read books all day. Balance is achieving our goals while enjoying the ride. It's being more deeply involved in our life but less attached. It's standing up for the life we want to live and making choices that align with that.

However, in our high-speed, high-pressure, high-stress world, balance is a challenge for most of us. It may be that we struggle to balance the demands of our career with a fulfilling social life. Or we could struggle to balance the needs of our young children with the need to look after our health. Or we might focus so much on serving others that we struggle to find the time to eat properly, exercise and rest.

I used to struggle a lot with finding balance and instead would take things to the extreme – extreme diets, extreme exercise plans, extreme working hours, extreme expectations, extreme highs and extreme lows. The truth is, extremes are easy but they take us out of balance. And when we are imbalanced, our body, mind and life suffers.

While finding balance is a fluid process, a lifetime project rather than a finite goal, chronic imbalance affects us physically, mentally and emotionally. Symptoms include anxiety, insecurity, loneliness, sadness, forgetfulness and a racing mind. We may suffer from bloating, aching joints, hot flushes, insomnia, overall fatigue and lack of vitality. Finding balance is a never-ending journey so what is important is learning how to recognise when we are slipping out of balance and having the courage to act in order to correct it.

Yoga is a wonderful way to bring our mind, body and spirit back into balance. It teaches us how to be both soft and strong. By using our breath and yoga poses we can practise finding balance on our yoga mat under the pressure of a deep backbend or while standing on one leg, which we can then use in everyday life.

Like yoga, Ayurveda is all about balance. It promotes health, happiness and personal growth through the proper balance of energies in the body using the external energy of things in our everyday life – food, exercise, the people we surround ourselves with, our work, and other lifestyle choices. For example, instead of focusing on following a 'balanced diet', we need to find a diet *that balances us*. If we are cold all the time, have dry skin and suffer from constipation, we need to include healthy oils and heating foods like spices in our diet. But if we are naturally hot all the time and have oily skin and we follow the same diet of oily, heating foods, we can suffer from acne, sweating and diarrhoea. This is why self-awareness (which we looked at on Day 1) and understanding our bodymind is so important for finding balance.

Likewise, Buddhism encourages us to take the middle path instead of falling into a cycle of extremes. The Buddhist attitude of equanimity teaches that true happiness comes from balance and not from dualities of pleasure and pain, gain and loss or rich and poor.

Heart-Centred Exploration

Being balanced doesn't mean that we feel calm, grounded and content all the time. Balance is a way of living – a practice that we need to explore every day. Some days we will find balance and feel centred, grounded and motivated, and some days we will lose it. The important thing is knowing how to find it again through our lifestyle choices.

Balance means different things to different people so today's exploration is about understanding what balance means to you.

Think of a time when you felt balanced – when you liked the way you looked, felt good about yourself as a person, and felt energised, centred and motivated. Now make a list of all the things that were going on in your life at the time. How did you spend your days? How long did you sleep for? What time did you go to bed? What time did you get up? What exercise did you do? What was your diet like? Who did you socialise with? How much time did you spend working? What hobbies did you have? How much time did you give to others? What books were you reading?

This list is a collection of things that keep you in balance. Keep hold of it and refer to it whenever you're feeling anxious or exhausted and alter your lifestyle by going to bed earlier, eating more vegetables, or spending more time doing whatever makes you feel grounded so that you can begin to bring your mind, body and life back into balance.

Finding Balance Sequence

Today's sequence uses a variety of standing, seated and inverted balances to help you feel grounded. Some of the poses are more challenging and you might wobble or fall, and that's OK. Sometimes balance means losing balance – for our passions and dreams and for those we love, so it's important we know how to rediscover our balance even if we have lost it for a little while.

Finding Balance Meditation

Practising balance means avoiding extremes. When it comes to our thoughts, memories and emotions, we often hold on to them and wallow in them or we shut off our hearts and avoid them completely. Today's meditation is called *'touch and go'*, and it helps us find balance by noticing whatever emotions arise and letting them go, instead of grabbing at them or pushing them away.

Find a comfortable seated position and focus on your breath. Begin by practising the extremes. Start with the *'touch and grab'* coping method. Notice whatever thought or emotion comes into your mind and focus on it, allowing a story to develop and letting yourself get sucked into the drama. After a couple of minutes, bring yourself out of the storyline and notice how you're feeling.

Now practise the other extreme – *'go and go'*. Let whatever thought or emotion arise, and ignore it by focusing on something else. Every time a feeling arises block it out by thinking of something else. It can help to think of a simple object like an animal or a piece of fruit, to distract you from whatever emotion arises. After a couple of minutes, reconnect with yourself.

Finally practise balance using *'touch and go'*. As a feeling arises, touch it gently by noticing it and engaging with the energy of the emotion for a moment without getting sucked into the story behind it. Allow yourself to feel whatever needs to be felt, and then let the feeling pass. Notice how much more balanced and grounded you feel when you allow yourself to experience emotions without avoidance or attachment.

Day 14: Finding Balance Sequence

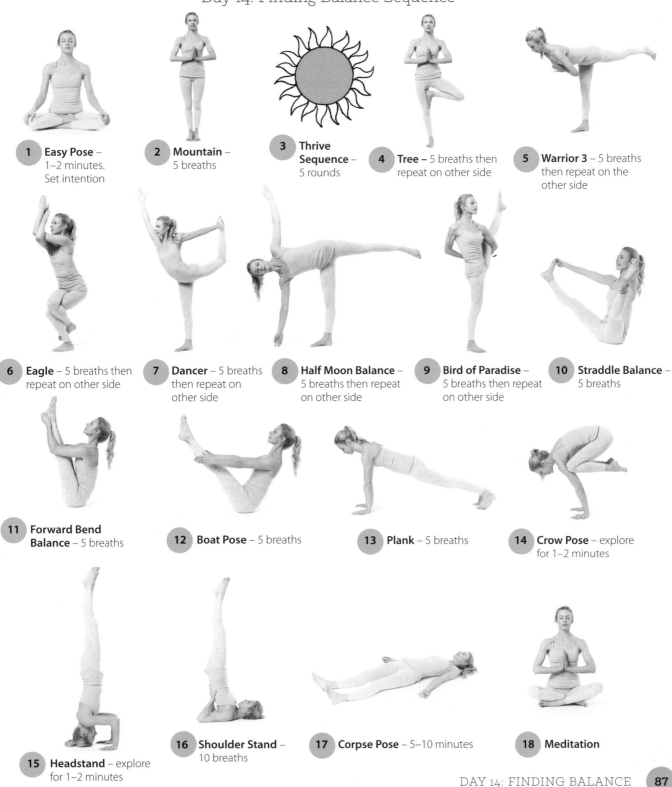

1 **Easy Pose** – 1–2 minutes. Set intention

2 **Mountain** – 5 breaths

3 **Thrive Sequence** – 5 rounds

4 **Tree** – 5 breaths then repeat on other side

5 **Warrior 3** – 5 breaths then repeat on the other side

6 **Eagle** – 5 breaths then repeat on other side

7 **Dancer** – 5 breaths then repeat on other side

8 **Half Moon Balance** – 5 breaths then repeat on other side

9 **Bird of Paradise** – 5 breaths then repeat on other side

10 **Straddle Balance** – 5 breaths

11 **Forward Bend Balance** – 5 breaths

12 **Boat Pose** – 5 breaths

13 **Plank** – 5 breaths

14 **Crow Pose** – explore for 1–2 minutes

15 **Headstand** – explore for 1–2 minutes

16 **Shoulder Stand** – 10 breaths

17 **Corpse Pose** – 5–10 minutes

18 **Meditation**

Day 15: Going with the Flow

Release your grip. Open your clenched fist.
Touch life. Don't strangle it.

Many us fight against the flow of life in an attempt to control the uncontrollables. We try to micromanage the universe to achieve the outcome we think is best for us. We waste precious energy planning and predicting things that we cannot possibly plan or predict.

In reality, life is a series of natural and spontaneous changes and when we try to control everything, we end up enjoying nothing. Worry never changes the outcome, but many of us spend our days in a state of stress and anxiety because we're so attached to a specific outcome – at work, in our relationships and of our diet. Whenever we feel under this sort of pressure it's because we have blocked the flow of life. It means we need to take a look at what expectations we can let go of so we can relax.

The struggles that many of us face on a daily basis – stress, anxiety and depression, may be normal in 21st-century life but they are not natural. If we take a look at nature itself we can see that life is not meant to be a struggle. The sun doesn't struggle to shine, birds don't struggle to fly and flowers don't struggle to bloom. When we force nothing, drop our expectations and relax into life, we turn off the furnace of struggle and begin to fully engage with the present moment and what we feel we are being called to do.

In the past I was a massive control freak. I tried to control everything from what and when I ate, to the number on the scale and the size of my thighs. Control is intricately related to disordered eating because food is something we can control when we feel like the rest of our life is in chaos. But my attempts to control food and my body never gave me the outcome that I wanted (freedom, love and happiness) and instead destroyed my health and blindfolded me to my intuition. Only when I did the opposite of controlling – surrendering – did I find the happiness I had been searching for. By surrendering to my appetite, my natural weight, spontaneous meals out and cake dates with friends, did I rediscover my passion for life.

Surrendering involves releasing the clenched fist we have around life. It means stopping fighting – with ourselves, with the universe and with the natural flow of things. When we are caught in the midst of a struggle we spend so much energy analysing the past, planning the future and trying to figure out how we feel and what we want. Sometimes the best thing to do is to surrender, embrace the uncertainty and see what happens.

When we embrace the flow of life there are fewer obstacles to deal with, our mind becomes clearer and we give ourselves the freedom to find our passion and purpose. Psychologists have identified 'flow' as a state of consciousness where we are so involved in whatever we are doing – a hobby, a relationship, or life in general, that we don't have enough attention left to notice any anxiety, distress or mental chatter. It is this flow state that redirects our energy away from worry and fear so that it can flow freely, that cultivates happiness. We can tell we're in a flow state when:

- We lose awareness of time and are completely present in whatever we are doing.
- We stop thinking about ourselves as we are so immersed in what we are doing that there is no room for thoughts, worries or self-consciousness.
- Our attention is razor sharp as all our mental resources are being channelled to the task at hand.
- Our work seems effortless despite being highly complex or requiring a great deal of mental effort.

Heart-Centred Exploration

Surrendering into the flow of life isn't always easy – especially if you've spent a long time trying to control every part of it. That is why it is important to practise surrendering so it is something that you can feel relaxed in doing. Today's exploration asks you to question: would letting go of control feel like freedom?

Start by pinpointing your fears so you can clear out your system a little. Take a notebook and write down the following headings: food; exercise; my body; my relationships; work; achievement; other people; other uncontrollables.

Under each heading write down:

- What are you afraid of?
- What's the worst that could happen if you don't control the outcome?
- Will each situation be worse if it doesn't work out the way you think it should? What other possible outcomes are there?
- Will letting go of control in each situation feel like freedom?

Going with the Flow Sequence

Today's sequence focuses on surrendering using a series of yin poses. By surrendering on our yoga mat we will learn how to surrender into the flow of life.

Going with the Flow Meditation

On Day 3 of our journey we focused on letting go of shame, fear and guilt. Today's meditation focuses on letting go of control – this is what we need to do so that we can go with the flow and relax into life.

The technique is simple, find a comfortable seated position and bring your awareness to your breath. As you inhale say to yourself *'let'* and as you exhale say *'go'.* As with the *'so'hum'* meditation we practised on Day 7, use the phrase 'let go' as a mantra to keep your focus in the moment, and help you block out any mental chatter and achieve the flow state. Stay here for 5–10 minutes until you feel calm and liberated, and return to this meditation any time you feel under pressure to remind you to release control and relax into life.

Day 15: Going with the Flow Sequence

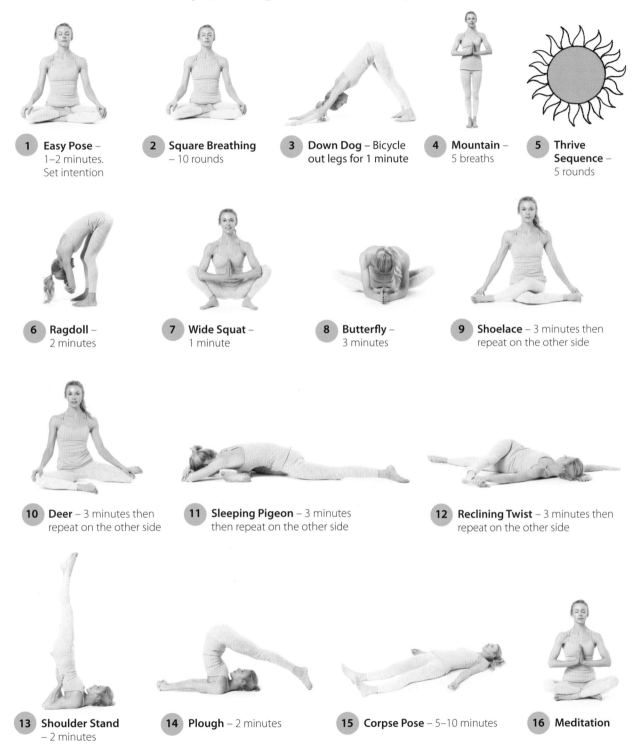

1 **Easy Pose** – 1–2 minutes. Set intention

2 **Square Breathing** – 10 rounds

3 **Down Dog** – Bicycle out legs for 1 minute

4 **Mountain** – 5 breaths

5 **Thrive Sequence** – 5 rounds

6 **Ragdoll** – 2 minutes

7 **Wide Squat** – 1 minute

8 **Butterfly** – 3 minutes

9 **Shoelace** – 3 minutes then repeat on the other side

10 **Deer** – 3 minutes then repeat on the other side

11 **Sleeping Pigeon** – 3 minutes then repeat on the other side

12 **Reclining Twist** – 3 minutes then repeat on the other side

13 **Shoulder Stand** – 2 minutes

14 **Plough** – 2 minutes

15 **Corpse Pose** – 5–10 minutes

16 **Meditation**

Day 16: Following Your Heart

Never let your ego silence your intuition. Never ignore the things that give you goosebumps. Never settle for mediocrity. Go after whatever sets you heart on fire.

· ·

What's in our heart is more important than what's in our bank account, job description or Facebook posts. Yet most of us spend more time and energy on money, work and social media than we do on the things that fill our hearts with magic and make us feel most alive.

Our culture is ego driven. We are taught to believe that happiness is based on success. This leaves us forever wanting a better job, bigger house and faster car. We want to be right. We want to be the best. We want it all. The problem with being driven by our ego is that we will never have it all. So we are left feeling increasingly dissatisfied with life.

An easy way to discover if we are being driven by our ego or following our heart is to ask ourselves whether we feel superior or inferior to others. If we feel either, then it is our ego that is in control and we are probably trapped in a cycle of comparison, fear and a constant need for approval.

The only way to escape this cycle is to follow our heart. This concept of following our heart is referred to as many things – quantum physics calls it energy, religion calls it spirit and psychology calls it intuition. It's the vibes, hunches and gut instincts we have that logic can't seem to explain. Science has found that when it comes to making major life decisions such as choosing a career path or who to marry, following our heart leads to better outcomes than trusting our logical thinking brain.

Despite this evidence, many of us struggle to follow our hearts because our ego interrupts our intuition. We doubt the vibes that come from our hearts because the messages are often based on facts just below the surface of consciousness. But our heart's desires are there for a reason. They are our *raison d'être* – our life's purpose and our reason for living. Even if they defy logic and upset our plans, we need to chase them so that we can find our purpose and feel truly alive.

I spent years being driven by my ego instead of following my heart. All of my childhood I dreamt of being a writer and teacher, but when I finished school and had to make decisions about my career, I did what I thought I had to do to be successful in life – I went to college, then university, and then did a Master's degree, all the time working in architects' offices and news agencies to build my CV and boost my bank balance. It was only when I was offered a PhD that I began to pay attention to my heart's calling. Just as I had used yoga to heal from anorexia and depression, I began to deepen my yoga practice and meditate more so I could tune back into my intuition and rediscover my passions. I turned down the PhD and found the courage to do the things that set my heart on fire – teach and write. Just two years later I had built a successful yoga business and had my first book published.

We betray ourselves when we do not follow our heart. When we have been detached from it for so long it can be difficult to stop our mental chatter and listen to what our heart has to say. One of the simplest ways to tune into our heart is to pay attention to what breaks it – that is our life's purpose. That is why I'm writing this book. Because my heart breaks a little bit every time I see someone with anorexia, or hear about someone's struggle with depression, or read about the 44 per cent of people suffering from stress and 27 per cent of people who admit to feeling close to breaking point. I am following my heart in the hope that it will illuminate the way for you to do the same.

Heart-Centred Exploration

Intuition and creativity are intimately related. Both connect us to our subconscious and help us move away from the control of our ego and towards the freedom and fulfilment that comes with following our heart.

Today's exploration is simple: do something creative. This could be painting a picture, baking a cake, listening to music, walking in nature, writing a poem or just allowing yourself to sit and day dream.

Follow Your Heart Sequence

In order to follow our heart, we need to release any blockages from it. Today's sequence focuses on our heart chakra so we can reconnect to our instincts and follow our dreams.

Heart Rhythm Meditation

Today's meditation is based around the concept of psychophysiological coherence. This is where our mind and body are working in harmony. We use our breathing to coordinate our body's various systems so there is unity between our heartbeat, our mind and our body.

Begin in a comfortable seated position and bring your awareness to your breath. As you breathe, pay attention to the centre of your chest, where your heart is, and imagine each breath flowing in and out of this area. Continue to breathe through your heart and begin to lengthen each exhalation for a count of six. After a few breaths, lengthen the inhalation for a count of six. After a few more breaths add in a pause at the top of the inhalation and the bottom of the exhalation. In these pauses bring your awareness to your heartbeat. The longer your hold your breath, the more your heartbeat will become clear. The clearer your awareness of your heartbeat is, the more you open up your consciousness and will be able to follow your heart.

Day 16: Follow Your Heart Sequence

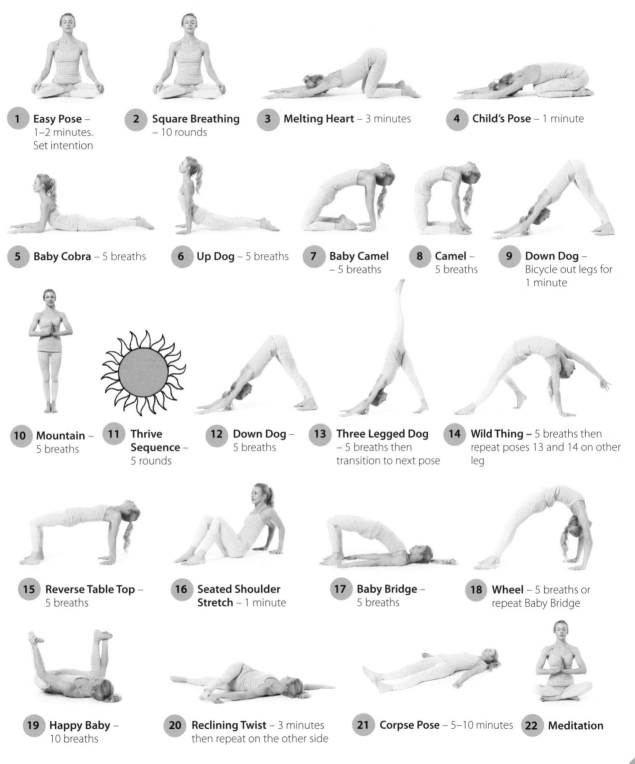

1 **Easy Pose** – 1–2 minutes. Set intention

2 **Square Breathing** – 10 rounds

3 **Melting Heart** – 3 minutes

4 **Child's Pose** – 1 minute

5 **Baby Cobra** – 5 breaths

6 **Up Dog** – 5 breaths

7 **Baby Camel** – 5 breaths

8 **Camel** – 5 breaths

9 **Down Dog** – Bicycle out legs for 1 minute

10 **Mountain** – 5 breaths

11 **Thrive Sequence** – 5 rounds

12 **Down Dog** – 5 breaths

13 **Three Legged Dog** – 5 breaths then transition to next pose

14 **Wild Thing** – 5 breaths then repeat poses 13 and 14 on other leg

15 **Reverse Table Top** – 5 breaths

16 **Seated Shoulder Stretch** – 1 minute

17 **Baby Bridge** – 5 breaths

18 **Wheel** – 5 breaths or repeat Baby Bridge

19 **Happy Baby** – 10 breaths

20 **Reclining Twist** – 3 minutes then repeat on the other side

21 **Corpse Pose** – 5–10 minutes

22 **Meditation**

Day 17: Embracing Discomfort

Every time we go through a period of transformation we will experience discomfort. But embracing this discomfort will bring us more happiness, love and freedom than our comfort zones ever will.

Discomfort is our compass towards thriving. It is the call to set ourselves free. It is in these moments of discomfort that we learn the most about ourselves so we can grow and evolve beyond the insecure person who continually seeks zones of comfort and instead begin to discover that we are strong enough to deal with whatever life throws at us.

Despite research showing that getting outside our comfort zone helps us perform better, be more creative and become the best version of ourselves, discomfort is still something many of us fear. For example, when it rains we tend to stay inside in the warmth instead of going out for a walk in the storm. By avoiding the discomfort of being cold, wet and weary, we miss out on the full texture of life. But what happens if the storm goes on for months and we run out of food? We have to venture outside of our comfort zone. In the same way the storm might not ease, the situation we are in might not change. So we need to.

Discomfort is not something we need to be afraid of. It is only when we are willing to stay with this uncomfortable energy that we gradually learn not to fear it. One of the biggest lessons I learnt on my journey through anorexia is that there is a big difference between wanting to change and being willing to change and experience the discomfort that comes with that change. I spent years wanting to recover but it was only when I was willing to experience the temporary discomfort that comes with eating more, gaining weight, and letting go of unhealthy habits that I found freedom.

Just like I turned to starvation and excessive exercise, many of us turn to shadow comforts in times of stress. These could be sugar, caffeine, alcohol, mindlessly watching TV or browsing social media – anything that helps us numb out, fill an empty space or gives us short-term satisfaction and relief. At some point we realise how these shadow comforts are keeping us trapped instead of helping us heal, so we begin to venture out of our comfort zone and explore healthier ways to face our fears and transcend our struggles.

It's this stage of discomfort that is the most challenging because we want to return to our comfort zone even though we know deep down that it is imprisoning us. I spent a long time in this in-between stage, wishing I could get the comfort I used to get from skipping meals and running until I was near collapse. But I quickly learnt that when life gets tough and someone we love dies or our relationship ends, the places we used to go for comfort – the daily glass of wine, weekend ice cream binge or wild night out partying, don't bring us comfort any more. Instead of finding another shadow comfort, repressing our discomfort or blaming someone else because we want a solution, it's staying in this in-between place that allows us to heal.

The truth is, leaving our comfort zone is hard. But staying in our comfort zone with our stress and our struggles is also hard. In order to thrive we need to have faith that thriving itself is possible so that we can choose courage over comfort and stay with whatever discomfort, emptiness or mess we are experiencing until we find peace and growth.

Heart-Centred Exploration

In order to embrace discomfort, we need to know what is outside of our comfort zone. And in order to do that we need to know what's inside it. Take a large piece of paper and draw a circle in the middle – this is your comfort zone. Inside this circle write all the day-to-day things that bring you comfort and make you feel safe. It can include your morning routine, your route to work, your lunch, your clothes, your books, your exercise class, the people you hang out with, where you sit in a café and what music you listen to.

Then outside of this circle write all the things that make you feel uncomfortable. This can range from simple things such as eating a new food or reading a different type of magazine, to travelling the world or telling someone you love them. Aim to write down 20–30 things that are outside of your comfort zone.

Once you have done this, place the piece of paper somewhere that is obvious for you to see and every day do one of the things you have written down that is outside of your comfort zone. Cook a new meal, cycle to work instead of walking, try a new exercise class, plan a date night, book that trip you've always wanted to take – keep exploring new things so that discomfort will no longer hold you back from experiencing life to the fullest.

Embracing Discomfort Sequence

Just like athletes embrace discomfort in their training so they grow stronger, in yoga we lean into any discomfort in each pose so that we learn not to fear it. One of the best ways of doing this is through playing our edge in yin yoga. Our edge refers to the edge of our comfort zone and we want to practise so that we are just outside of it – far enough so we feel the pose working but not so far that we feel pain. We want to play this edge so that as our body begins to release into the pose and our comfort zone grows we move deeper into it to keep our bodymind strengthening and opening.

Embracing Discomfort Meditation

Meditation is a beautiful way to embrace discomfort because it gives us an opportunity to experience slight discomfort and learn to be with it.

Begin in a seated position and close your eyes. Focus on your breath for as long as you can. The first time you feel the urge to reposition yourself, open your eyes or get on with your day, resist it and stay focused on your breath. The second time you feel your body getting uncomfortable with the position you are sat in, or your mind getting uncomfortable with the process of focusing on your breath, resist the urge to move and keep focusing on your breathing. The third time you feel discomfort wave over you, allow yourself to fidget, open your eyes or end the meditation and gently carry on with your day. Over time this will help you learn to be with discomfort, instead of running from it every time you experience anxiety or distress.

Day 17: Embracing Discomfort Sequence

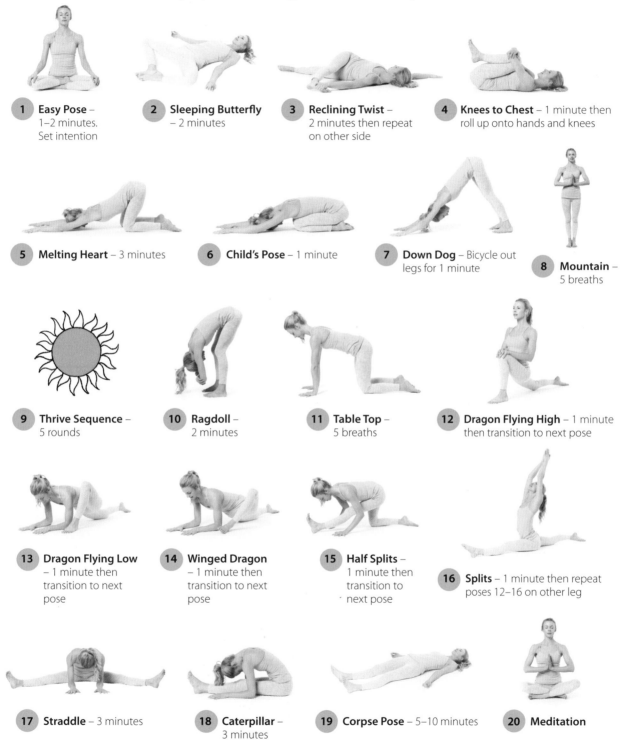

1 **Easy Pose** – 1–2 minutes. Set intention

2 **Sleeping Butterfly** – 2 minutes

3 **Reclining Twist** – 2 minutes then repeat on other side

4 **Knees to Chest** – 1 minute then roll up onto hands and knees

5 **Melting Heart** – 3 minutes

6 **Child's Pose** – 1 minute

7 **Down Dog** – Bicycle out legs for 1 minute

8 **Mountain** – 5 breaths

9 **Thrive Sequence** – 5 rounds

10 **Ragdoll** – 2 minutes

11 **Table Top** – 5 breaths

12 **Dragon Flying High** – 1 minute then transition to next pose

13 **Dragon Flying Low** – 1 minute then transition to next pose

14 **Winged Dragon** – 1 minute then transition to next pose

15 **Half Splits** – 1 minute then transition to next pose

16 **Splits** – 1 minute then repeat poses 12–16 on other leg

17 **Straddle** – 3 minutes

18 **Caterpillar** – 3 minutes

19 **Corpse Pose** – 5–10 minutes

20 **Meditation**

Day 18:
Being
Vulnerable

There is nothing so utterly terrifying and beautifully rewarding as being completely vulnerable. When you are courageous enough to take off your mask, you will find freedom, you will find connection, you will find yourself.

We are born in a state of vulnerability. We need food, water, shelter and love. We cry when we need to, eat when we are hungry and share our love fearlessly and unconditionally. Then somewhere along the way to adulthood we learn to hide our vulnerability, shut our emotions off and only share certain parts of ourselves with the world.

Social media epitomises our invulnerability. We share carefully calculated snippets of our lives with followers while sometimes shutting real people – our friends, partners and family, out of our day-to-day life. We edit, filter and Photoshop each post to add another layer of armour and further cement our masks because we fear that being our true selves is not good enough.

We all wear masks. Masks of make-up, muscle and money that hide our fears, failures and flaws. We wear masks to be the perfect parent, partner or child. We wear them to protect us from heartbreak and to hide ourselves because we're afraid that if people were to see the real us – with all our imperfections and struggles, they will no longer love us.

But wearing a mask is exhausting. Trust me, I wore one for years. Anorexia was my mask, my armour. It separated me from the world, numbed me from my feelings, and allowed me to avoid the vulnerability that comes with connection and intimacy. But after a while the armour got too heavy and I realised that the only way for me to be free from my struggles was to be vulnerable – to risk being rejected and misunderstood and expose my broken, fragmented, confused self to the world.

There can be no vulnerability without risk. The courage it takes to reveal ourselves fully is one of the most terrifying experiences in life but it will set us free. When we rip off our masks, discard our armour, and choose a raw and unguarded way of living we allow others to do the same. By doing this, we form deep, meaningful, soul connections that truly nourish us.

The power of vulnerability has become more widespread thanks to the work of researcher and storyteller Brené Brown. In a TED talk that has been watched over 30 million times, she cites vulnerability as the origin of creativity, innovation, change, joy, faith and connection. Vulnerability includes:

- Asking for what we need.
- Talking about how we're feeling.
- Having the hard conversations.
- Choosing to be authentic.
- Giving and receiving without judgement.
- Revealing our heart.
- Showing up even when we have no control over the outcome.

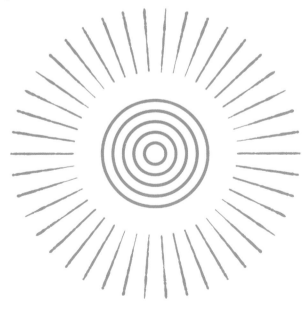

Heart-Centred Exploration

Like gratitude, vulnerability is a daily practice. A big part of vulnerability is honesty – with yourself and with others. Today's exploration asks you to be vulnerable and honest with someone close to you by asking for help.

A big sign that you are wearing a mask is that you think you need to do everything by yourself all the time for fear of being judged a failure. Asking for help involves admitting your weaknesses but, in doing so, you create space for connection by allowing others to share their strengths with you.

Write a list of all the things you would like help with and who you would like that help from but are too afraid to ask. It can be little things like wanting your partner to help with cleaning the bathroom or a work colleague to help out on a project. Or it could be a more life-changing thing like wanting support recovering from depression by asking a friend to go with you to a self-help group. Now number these things in order of what you would find the easiest to ask for help to the hardest. Today, ask for help with the first thing on your list and work your way through the list each day so you feel more confident being vulnerable and taking off your mask.

Vulnerability Sequence

Vulnerability relates to several of our chakras, mainly our pelvic chakra through the relationship of power and vulnerability, and the throat chakra through self-expression and being vulnerable enough to speak out truthfully. Today's sequence focuses on opening both chakras through hip openers and backbends to release blockages that may be contributing towards our resistance to reveal ourselves fully.

Vulnerability Meditation

There is something about eye contact that makes us feel vulnerable. Many of us end up avoiding it out of fear we are being judged, or just because we feel awkward. However, eye contact is one of the best ways to develop a soul-to-soul connection, and eye gazing is a beautiful meditation practice to find the courage to do this in everyday life.

Eye gazing is a traditional practice in both Buddhist and Hindu traditions and research has found that the more we gaze into another's eyes, the more connection and love we feel for them.

There are two options for today's meditation depending on whether you want to explore it with someone close to you or on your own.

Option one is to ask someone close to you to join you and begin by sitting comfortably opposite each other. Gaze gently and deeply into each other's eyes for five minutes, allowing any thoughts or worries to pass effortlessly by bringing your focus back to your partner's eyes. If this seems too much, then option two is to do the same meditation but this time gaze into your own eyes in a mirror for five minutes and begin to let your guard down and connect with your raw and unguarded self.

Day 18: Vulnerable Sequence

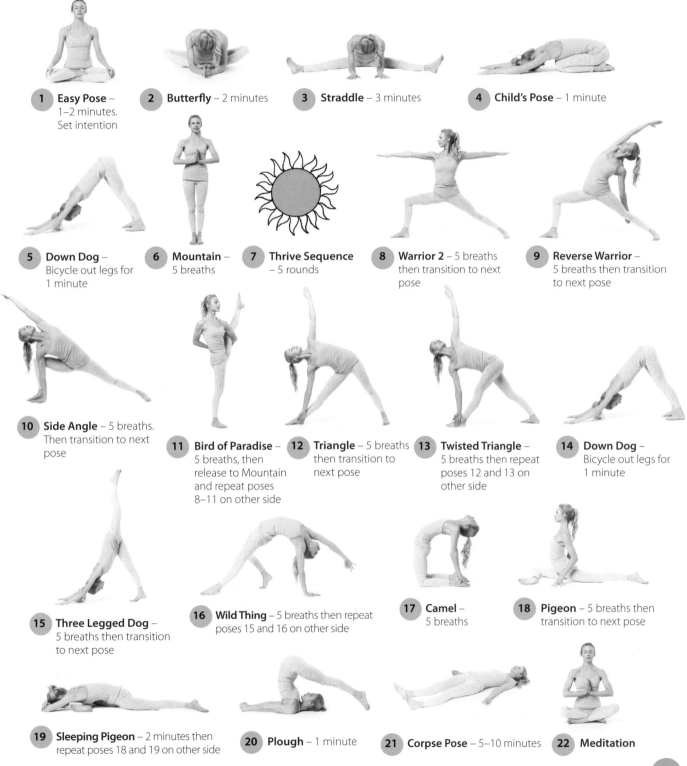

1 **Easy Pose** – 1–2 minutes. Set intention

2 **Butterfly** – 2 minutes

3 **Straddle** – 3 minutes

4 **Child's Pose** – 1 minute

5 **Down Dog** – Bicycle out legs for 1 minute

6 **Mountain** – 5 breaths

7 **Thrive Sequence** – 5 rounds

8 **Warrior 2** – 5 breaths then transition to next pose

9 **Reverse Warrior** – 5 breaths then transition to next pose

10 **Side Angle** – 5 breaths. Then transition to next pose

11 **Bird of Paradise** – 5 breaths, then release to Mountain and repeat poses 8–11 on other side

12 **Triangle** – 5 breaths then transition to next pose

13 **Twisted Triangle** – 5 breaths then repeat poses 12 and 13 on other side

14 **Down Dog** – Bicycle out legs for 1 minute

15 **Three Legged Dog** – 5 breaths then transition to next pose

16 **Wild Thing** – 5 breaths then repeat poses 15 and 16 on other side

17 **Camel** – 5 breaths

18 **Pigeon** – 5 breaths then transition to next pose

19 **Sleeping Pigeon** – 2 minutes then repeat poses 18 and 19 on other side

20 **Plough** – 1 minute

21 **Corpse Pose** – 5–10 minutes

22 **Meditation**

Day 19: Choosing to Love

Love changes everything. Choose it.
And use it to transform the world.

Love is the most healing force there is. Unfortunately, many of us struggle to love ourselves. We struggle to love the real, imperfect, beautifully flawed, slightly weird, magical people we are. We place conditions on our love – that we'll love ourselves when we lose weight, get a promotion, become a better person, stop drinking so much, get a boyfriend, or whatever other prerequisites we place on giving and receiving love.

The truth is, loving ourselves is not the result of thriving. Loving ourselves is the route to thriving. And it is a choice. Just like we can choose anger, sadness or hate, we can choose love. But in order to do this, in order to truly love ourselves, we cannot hate the experiences that shaped us. That is where many of us struggle with self-love. For some reason we believe that if we shame ourselves, we will end up loving ourselves. Shame never leads to love. Only love leads to love.

Loving ourselves isn't just an idea or a feeling. It involves action. Even if we are struggling to love ourselves, we can choose to act as if we do – to eat like we love ourselves, move like we love ourselves, talk like we love ourselves, and live every day like we love ourselves. Once we bring love into our daily life, we begin to realise its true power.

Through all the struggles I've been through in life, it wasn't the money in my bank or stamps on my passport that made me feel whole. It wasn't the beauty of my boyfriend or the number of exams I passed that made me feel at peace. Being a good weightlifter, strong yogi or successful author didn't give me the strength to face life's challenges. I got through anorexia, depression, anxiety, pain and sadness because of love.

Our possessions, accomplishments, titles, medals and money all pale into insignificance when we are faced with struggle. It is only love that will nurture us back when we are sick, heal us when we are grieving and rebuild us when our heart has been broken.

When we take a step back from our everyday struggles it's obvious that the thing that matters most is love. It doesn't matter what our body looks like, how successful our career is, how advanced our yoga practice is, how big our house is or what our bank statement says. The only thing that matters is how much we love – ourselves, other people and the world.

It is impossible to truly love others if we don't love ourselves. By choosing to love within, we learn to love the world. By learning to love the world, we discover there is something within us that the world needs. No matter how overwhelming our struggles may be right now, we can make a difference in the world. Through love, we discover new purpose and new meaning in our lives. We thrive.

Heart-Centred Exploration

Loving ourselves involves a deep appreciation for who we are. This isn't a feeling we have to conjure up but actions we can take. Today's exploration is simple. Ask yourself the question: *what can I do to love myself?*

Make a list of all the actions you can take to love yourself. This might include eating wholesome, nourishing food instead of skipping meals or bingeing on takeaways. It might involve going on a daily walk around the park every evening instead of watching a depressing soap on TV. Or it might include saying 'no' to other people for a while so you can rest and restore your energy. Aim to write 10 actions you can take to love yourself and incorporate them into your everyday life.

Choose Love Sequence

This heart-centred sequence helps you bring meditation into your yoga practice by asking you to put the emotions and sensations you feel in each pose into words. These can include physical sensations such as *'tight'*, *'tense'* and *'tired'*, as well as feelings and emotions such as *'anxious'*, *'sad'* and *'angry'*. As you acknowledge and experience each emotion instead of running away from them, you will find you'll be able to let them go and create space for love.

Love Yourself Meditation

Today's meditation helps you love yourself unconditionally by imagining that your personality is a child and you are its parent. By observing yourself from the perspective of someone who enjoys watching you grow and loves you unconditionally, you will begin to see yourself as someone intrinsically worthy of your own love.

Begin in a comfortable seated position, close your eyes and bring your awareness to your breath. Take some time to reflect on your personality including your traits, strengths, weaknesses and characteristics. Now imagine that your personality is your child and you are its parent. Notice how your thoughts and feelings about your personality change when you see it as a child – how you forgive its mistakes, accept its flaws and see its potential for growth. Notice the compassion you feel towards your child and then embrace it with unconditional love.

Bring this element of unconditional love into your everyday life. Every time you notice a lack of self-love in your life, see yourself as the child and remind yourself of the compassion, forgiveness and acceptance you deserve.

Day 19: Choose Love Sequence

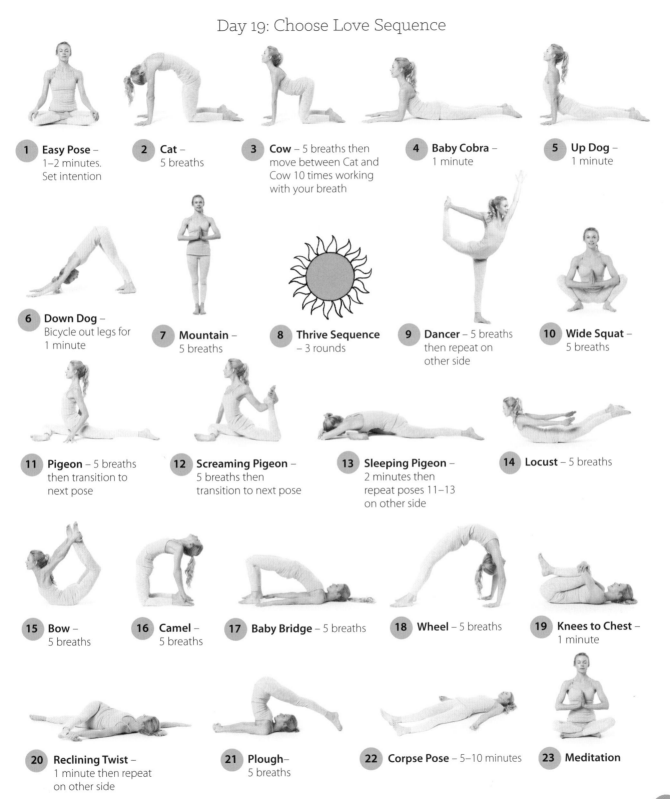

1 **Easy Pose** – 1–2 minutes. Set intention

2 **Cat** – 5 breaths

3 **Cow** – 5 breaths then move between Cat and Cow 10 times working with your breath

4 **Baby Cobra** – 1 minute

5 **Up Dog** – 1 minute

6 **Down Dog** – Bicycle out legs for 1 minute

7 **Mountain** – 5 breaths

8 **Thrive Sequence** – 3 rounds

9 **Dancer** – 5 breaths then repeat on other side

10 **Wide Squat** – 5 breaths

11 **Pigeon** – 5 breaths then transition to next pose

12 **Screaming Pigeon** – 5 breaths then transition to next pose

13 **Sleeping Pigeon** – 2 minutes then repeat poses 11–13 on other side

14 **Locust** – 5 breaths

15 **Bow** – 5 breaths

16 **Camel** – 5 breaths

17 **Baby Bridge** – 5 breaths

18 **Wheel** – 5 breaths

19 **Knees to Chest** – 1 minute

20 **Reclining Twist** – 1 minute then repeat on other side

21 **Plough** – 5 breaths

22 **Corpse Pose** – 5–10 minutes

23 **Meditation**

Day 20: Re-Authoring Your Life Story

Don't be ashamed of your story. People are hungry for it. It isn't perfect. But it's wild. It's passionate. It's courageous. Owning it will help you heal. And sharing it will help heal the world.

Stories are an intrinsic part of our life. They are one of the things that make us human. From the bedtime fairy tales our parents read to us as children to the movies we watch, the music we listen to and the news we follow, storytelling influences all aspects of our life. And no stories influence our values, desires, dreams and beliefs more than the stories we tell ourselves.

These stories can empower us to chase our dreams or they can trap us in a cycle of destructive behaviour. We live the stories we tell ourselves as if they are true. This means that we cannot thrive if we keep telling ourselves stories which break us down and cause us pain. We need to listen to the stories we tell ourselves and open up to new ways of looking at our experiences, so we can reconstruct an understanding of who we are and our place in the world.

We are the author of our life story. We create it from the meanings we make from every aspect of our lives. When the meanings we make are negative we end up disempowering ourselves with limiting beliefs of inadequacy, stupidity and hopelessness. We find that every thought, word and action is driven by our struggles – we become attached to our story and forget that we can write a new chapter any time we choose.

There is a difference between owning our story and being attached to and trapped by it. When we are imprisoned by our story we defend our victimhood, blame the past for our current struggles and feel shame, regret and totally powerless to change. However, when we own our story we give ourselves the power to change it – to interpret every experience in a way that empowers us and leads to more joy, more connection and more fulfilment. By changing our story, we change our life.

It has taken me a long time to not be ashamed of my story. I didn't talk about my struggle with anorexia and depression for years because I hoped that not talking about the pain would mean I wouldn't feel it. But when we deny our story, it ends up defining us. I couldn't find freedom because I always felt I had something to hide. It was only when I found the courage to own my story – the beautiful, the wild and the messy parts, that I began to free myself to write a brave new ending.

Psychologists often call our life stories schemas or cognitive maps, and these schemas direct what we notice, how we interpret things, how we make decisions, how we act and how we see ourselves. Researchers have found that when we have a schema where we see ourselves as victims and the world is unsafe, we end up with high levels of distress, but when we have stories in which we view ourselves as survivors or thrivers, we heal and grow.

Thriving isn't about being fixed (we were never broken) – it's about deconstructing our life story, while reconstructing a new one with a new understanding of how our struggles have transformed us. Professor Stephen Joseph, an expert in thriving, explains that it is meaning that provides us with the strength to move forward. So, by giving our struggles meaning in the story of our life, we create a sense of purpose, connection and fulfilment.

Heart-Centred Exploration

Re-authoring our life story begins by how we look at ourselves in relation to our struggles. Do we see ourselves as passive, helpless victims? As survivors who recognise the struggles we have been through? Or as thrivers who are moving beyond our struggles to find meaning and purpose in our lives.

Today's exploration involves understanding how you view yourself in your life story by reflecting on the words you use. Below are three lists of words associated with being a victim, survivor and thriver. Spend 5–10 minutes adding as many words as you can to each list. Once you've finished, reflect on which words you use the most in your thoughts and speech and work towards using more of the words related to thriving in your everyday life.

Victim	**Survivor**	**Thriver**
Blame	Endure	Hopeful
Destruction	Exist	Fulfilment
Powerless	Fighter	Meaning
Sacrifice	Persevere	Purpose
Suffer	Recognise	Resilience
Underdog	Tolerate	Responsibility

Re-Authoring Sequence

Today's sequence uses lots of standing poses including the Warrior series, because it's hard to feel like a victim when you're in strong and empowering poses like these.

Re-Authoring Meditation

Today's meditation is a walking meditation. This represents finding freedom from any disempowering stories and walking away from destructive habits. Ideally find somewhere to walk that is surrounded by nature – a field, a woodland or a park. You don't need to walk far: 10 to 20 minutes will be enough time for you to use the physical, mental and emotional experience of walking to feel the freedom that comes with moving forwards in life.

As you begin walking focus on your body, starting at the soles of your feet and noticing how each heel and ball of the foot make contact with the ground. Draw your focus up your legs to your ankles, calves, knees and thighs, noticing how each muscle contracts and relaxes to move the body part. Become aware of your hips, your belly, your spine and your upper body. Once you've scanned your whole body, bring your awareness to any feelings or emotions – noticing them and letting them go without getting caught up in any stories. Then see if you can find a balance of awareness between the outer bodily sensations and inner feelings.

This walking meditation will help you bring your meditation practice into the outside world.

Day 20: Re-Authoring Sequence

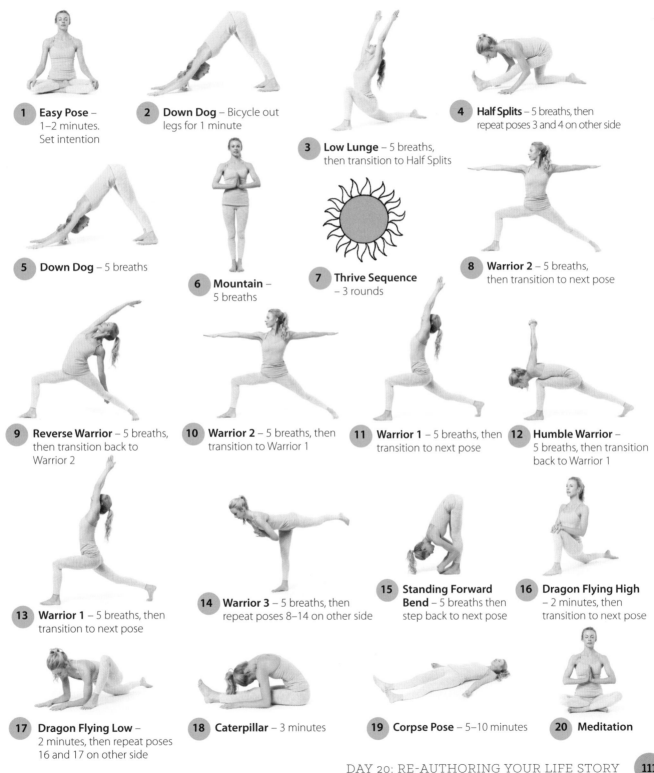

1 **Easy Pose** – 1–2 minutes. Set intention

2 **Down Dog** – Bicycle out legs for 1 minute

3 **Low Lunge** – 5 breaths, then transition to Half Splits

4 **Half Splits** – 5 breaths, then repeat poses 3 and 4 on other side

5 **Down Dog** – 5 breaths

6 **Mountain** – 5 breaths

7 **Thrive Sequence** – 3 rounds

8 **Warrior 2** – 5 breaths, then transition to next pose

9 **Reverse Warrior** – 5 breaths, then transition back to Warrior 2

10 **Warrior 2** – 5 breaths, then transition to Warrior 1

11 **Warrior 1** – 5 breaths, then transition to next pose

12 **Humble Warrior** – 5 breaths, then transition back to Warrior 1

13 **Warrior 1** – 5 breaths, then transition to next pose

14 **Warrior 3** – 5 breaths, then repeat poses 8–14 on other side

15 **Standing Forward Bend** – 5 breaths then step back to next pose

16 **Dragon Flying High** – 2 minutes, then transition to next pose

17 **Dragon Flying Low** – 2 minutes, then repeat poses 16 and 17 on other side

18 **Caterpillar** – 3 minutes

19 **Corpse Pose** – 5–10 minutes

20 **Meditation**

Day 21: Transforming Yourself and the World

Transformation is often more about unlearning than learning. Unbecoming before becoming. Unlosing and losing yourself over and over again so that you can be the totally real, beautifully raw, and uniquely magical you. Because the world needs that. The world needs YOU.

If we transform ourselves, we can transform our world. If we can transform our inner world and forgive ourselves, soften our hearts and grow stronger, wiser and more compassionate, then our outer world will transform too.

The difficult thing with transformation is that it is tough. We think of it like emerging as the butterfly, when in reality it is the messy work of pushing out the cocoon. It can be dark and painful as we come to face our demons and everything in our life begins to shift. Some periods of transformation are so confusing that it is difficult to see that growth is happening at all. This is because whenever we go through a phase of personal growth we tend to feel it through hurt, hate or heartache. It can feel like we're breaking or falling apart, but that brokenness gives birth to a new way of loving, accepting and relating to the world. It creates space for us to grow into something different with a new capacity to become the person we want to become.

One of the hardest lessons I've learnt on my journey is that transformation involves loss. Any time we grow, we are going to lose something – identities, relationships, habits, belief systems, the things that make us feel comfortable.

When I decided to find freedom from anorexia, I grieved for the loss of the scared, insecure, emaciated person that I had been even though I no longer wanted to be her. I grieved for the loss of comfort I found in starvation and for the loss of satisfaction I found when the scales went down. When I turned down a PhD and walked away from a career in academia, I grieved for the loss of my academic self even though I knew it wouldn't give me purpose or fulfilment. And when my ex-boyfriend and I decided to end our relationship, I grieved for the loss of a future I had imagined we would share, even though I knew we had outgrown each other. But loss creates space. As old energy clears out, we allow new energy to enter. We create room for new people, adventures and experiences in our lives.

As we transform ourselves on a personal level, we begin to see life in a new light. We make choices and take actions we never would have thought of taking had we been stuck in old habits and thought patterns. This is how we change the world. As soon as we believe that we are important and our life matters, we recognise that every individual is important and every life matters. We don't have to move mountains or revolutionise the world single-handedly. We can transform our lives and the lives of others just by living with acceptance, gratitude and an unshakeable belief in the power of kindness, compassion and love.

As we come to the end of our journey together, and you continue your adventure towards thriving, I want you to remember that the struggles we experience at certain points in our lives do not make us helpless victims of lifelong conditions. Things don't always go to plan and broken things don't always get fixed, but if we continue to love and we continue to forgive, we will continue to thrive.

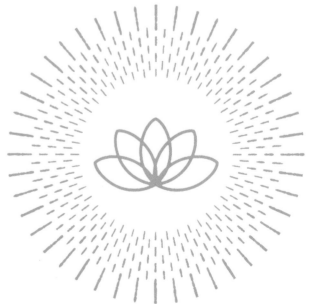

Heart-Centred Exploration

One of the simplest and most beautiful ways to transform yourself and the world is one simple act of kindness at a time. Usually this involves helping someone, complimenting someone or thanking someone. It doesn't have to be a big thing. Common acts of kindness include: saying good morning to a stranger as you walk down the street, offering to pick up shopping for an elderly neighbour, holding the door open for someone, donating your old clothes to charity, bringing a cup of coffee to your assistant at work, sending flowers to a friend going through a hard time, doing the washing up for your family, passing on a brilliant book when you've finished reading it, or really listening to someone who needs to open their heart to you.

Kindness is contagious. Just like throwing a pebble into a pond and watching the ripples spread outwards, your single act of kind-heartedness will ripple and radiate into the world. Never underestimate the impact of a simple act of kindness.

Transformation Sequence

Yoga is a powerful route to transformation because it connects us to our intuition. This gives us access to our deepest desires and provides us with the inspiration to live the life we dream of. Today's sequence gives you a basic outline for your practice and asks you to tap into your intuition to create a practice that is right for you in this moment. Adjust it depending on how you feel physically and energetically and what intention you have as you step on your mat.

Transformation Meditation

Meditation is not just for our own benefit. We want whatever we learn while meditating to be of use so that we can serve others and so that others get the best of us. This means integrating our meditation into our everyday life – meditation in action. This can take years of practice as it means being able to meditate on the world while also functioning in it. It means that each experience we encounter can bring us into a deeper meditative space. This space allows us to stay quiet inside each time we observe, respond and act in our everyday lives so that we can live consciously instead of out of habit.

Experiment with meditation in action over the next few days, weeks and years. As you walk focus on your breath, as you eat be aware of any mental chatter, and as you interact notice where your mind is wandering. Instead of getting pulled in the directions of anxiety, desire and fear, do your best to stay in your meditative space so that you can see each experience as an opportunity to thrive.

Day 21: Transformation Sequence

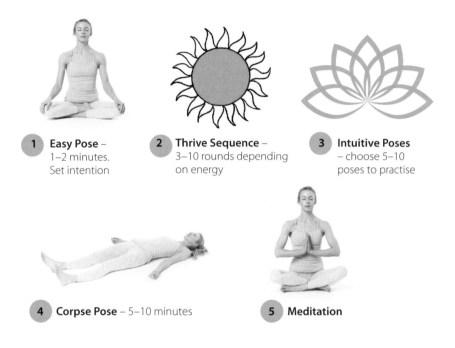

1. **Easy Pose** – 1–2 minutes. Set intention

2. **Thrive Sequence** – 3–10 rounds depending on energy

3. **Intuitive Poses** – choose 5–10 poses to practise

4. **Corpse Pose** – 5–10 minutes

5. **Meditation**

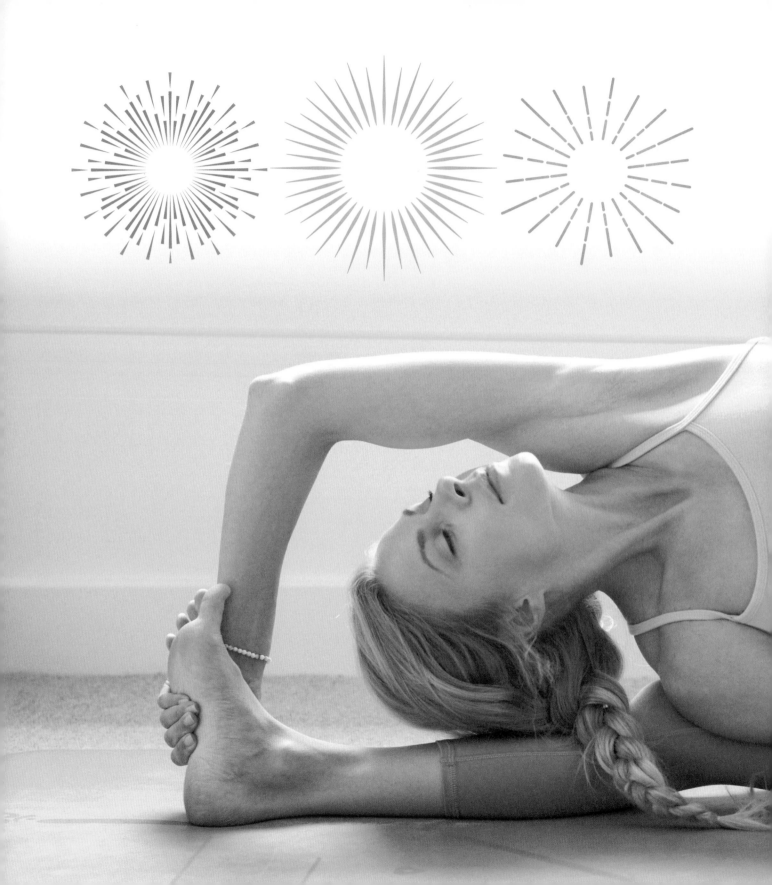

Part 4: Sequences to Help You Thrive

Yoga can be especially helpful at times in our lives when we are really struggling. This includes intense moments of anxiety or depression, when we're struggling to sleep or lacking in energy, and when we're feeling any body shame or lack of love for our body. The following five sequences are for you to use in these moments. Each sequence focuses on certain muscles and chakras and uses a specific combination of poses that will help ease that particular struggle.

Yoga for Easing Anxiety

Yoga helps ease anxiety by teaching us to stay in the present moment. By focusing on our breath and how our body feels in each pose, we keep ourselves anchored in the present so we can lower our emotional arousal and, instead of reacting fearfully to worries and anxious thoughts, we can acknowledge them with curiosity, and then let them go. This sequence focuses on releasing stress from the muscles that commonly tense up when we are anxious to create a sense of stillness and calm in your bodymind.

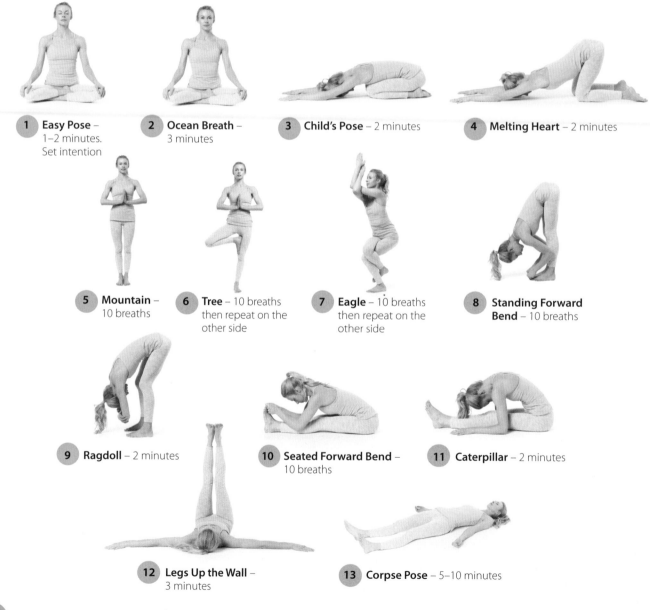

1 **Easy Pose** – 1–2 minutes. Set intention

2 **Ocean Breath** – 3 minutes

3 **Child's Pose** – 2 minutes

4 **Melting Heart** – 2 minutes

5 **Mountain** – 10 breaths

6 **Tree** – 10 breaths then repeat on the other side

7 **Eagle** – 10 breaths then repeat on the other side

8 **Standing Forward Bend** – 10 breaths

9 **Ragdoll** – 2 minutes

10 **Seated Forward Bend** – 10 breaths

11 **Caterpillar** – 2 minutes

12 **Legs Up the Wall** – 3 minutes

13 **Corpse Pose** – 5–10 minutes

Yoga for Relieving Depression

Yoga helps relieve depression by increasing levels of the neurotransmitter gamma-aminobutyric acid (GABA) in the brain. People experiencing depression tend to have lower levels of GABA and research shows that yoga increases this neurotransmitter, helping us feel calm and relaxed. Research also shows that emotions such as depression can affect the way our heart functions so this sequence focuses on releasing tension from the area around our chest to release stress, improve our posture and boost our mood.

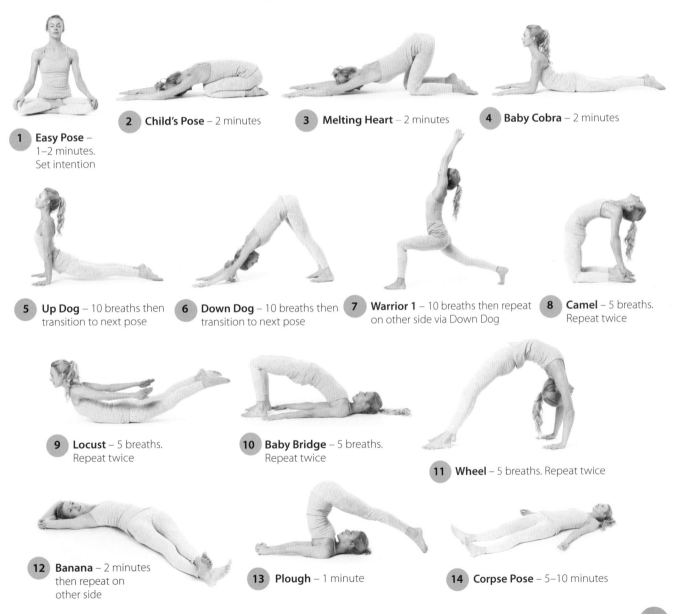

1 **Easy Pose** – 1–2 minutes. Set intention

2 **Child's Pose** – 2 minutes

3 **Melting Heart** – 2 minutes

4 **Baby Cobra** – 2 minutes

5 **Up Dog** – 10 breaths then transition to next pose

6 **Down Dog** – 10 breaths then transition to next pose

7 **Warrior 1** – 10 breaths then repeat on other side via Down Dog

8 **Camel** – 5 breaths. Repeat twice

9 **Locust** – 5 breaths. Repeat twice

10 **Baby Bridge** – 5 breaths. Repeat twice

11 **Wheel** – 5 breaths. Repeat twice

12 **Banana** – 2 minutes then repeat on other side

13 **Plough** – 1 minute

14 **Corpse Pose** – 5–10 minutes

Yoga for Boosting Body Image

Yoga provides us with a new way to relate to our body. Instead of judging it for what it looks like, we can draw our awareness inwards and connect to how it feels to live in our body. Where do I feel tight? Where am I holding tension? Where am I open? How can I release this discomfort? How does it feel to move through each pose? This gives us a new way to experience our body off the mat so we begin to nourish it instead of punish it. Poor body image can leave us feeling unstable so this sequence uses grounding poses to create a sense of strength, stability and courage.

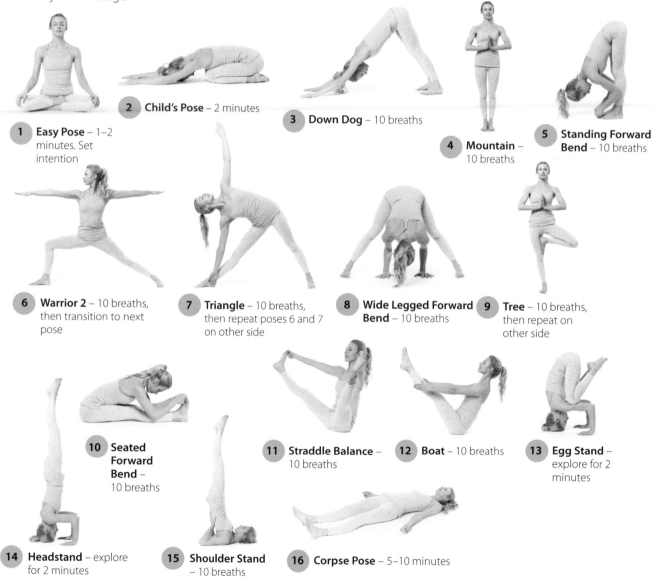

1 **Easy Pose** – 1–2 minutes. Set intention

2 **Child's Pose** – 2 minutes

3 **Down Dog** – 10 breaths

4 **Mountain** – 10 breaths

5 **Standing Forward Bend** – 10 breaths

6 **Warrior 2** – 10 breaths, then transition to next pose

7 **Triangle** – 10 breaths, then repeat poses 6 and 7 on other side

8 **Wide Legged Forward Bend** – 10 breaths

9 **Tree** – 10 breaths, then repeat on other side

10 **Seated Forward Bend** – 10 breaths

11 **Straddle Balance** – 10 breaths

12 **Boat** – 10 breaths

13 **Egg Stand** – explore for 2 minutes

14 **Headstand** – explore for 2 minutes

15 **Shoulder Stand** – 10 breaths

16 **Corpse Pose** – 5–10 minutes

Yoga to Help You Sleep

Yoga helps us get a peaceful night's sleep by calming our mind, releasing physical tension and activating our parasympathetic nervous system (the part of our nervous system responsible for rest, relaxation and digestion). Research has found that yoga reduces insomnia, so this sequence is a beautiful way to soothe our body and mind before we go to sleep – you can even practise it in bed!

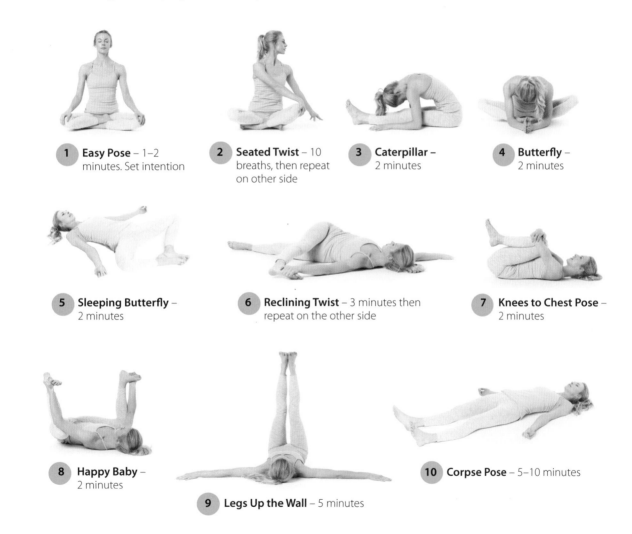

1 **Easy Pose** – 1–2 minutes. Set intention

2 **Seated Twist** – 10 breaths, then repeat on other side

3 **Caterpillar** – 2 minutes

4 **Butterfly** – 2 minutes

5 **Sleeping Butterfly** – 2 minutes

6 **Reclining Twist** – 3 minutes then repeat on the other side

7 **Knees to Chest Pose** – 2 minutes

8 **Happy Baby** – 2 minutes

9 **Legs Up the Wall** – 5 minutes

10 **Corpse Pose** – 5–10 minutes

Yoga to Increase Energy

Yoga helps to reduce fatigue and leave us feeling revitalised by unblocking stuck energy in our body. By moving the body we're waking up our nervous and circulatory systems so we feel more awake and energised. This sequence focuses on opening up the body and elongating the spine to release any blocked energy and help us feel more alive.

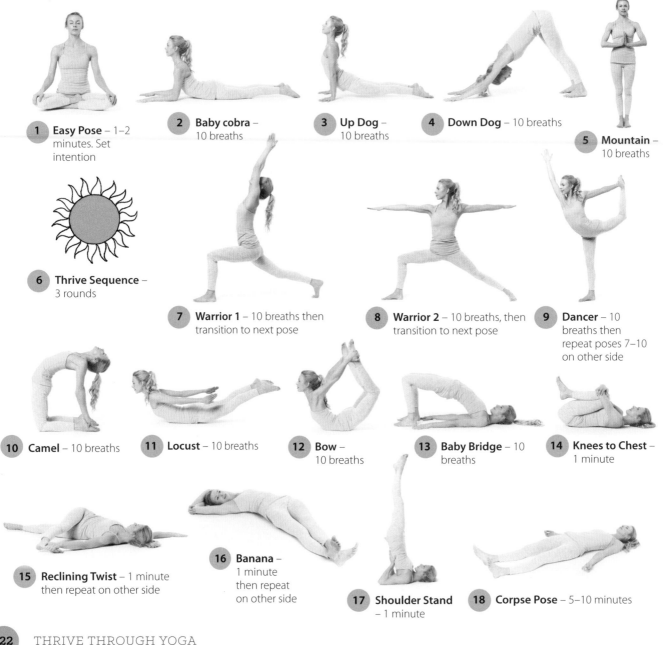

1 **Easy Pose** – 1–2 minutes. Set intention

2 **Baby cobra** – 10 breaths

3 **Up Dog** – 10 breaths

4 **Down Dog** – 10 breaths

5 **Mountain** – 10 breaths

6 **Thrive Sequence** – 3 rounds

7 **Warrior 1** – 10 breaths then transition to next pose

8 **Warrior 2** – 10 breaths, then transition to next pose

9 **Dancer** – 10 breaths then repeat poses 7–10 on other side

10 **Camel** – 10 breaths

11 **Locust** – 10 breaths

12 **Bow** – 10 breaths

13 **Baby Bridge** – 10 breaths

14 **Knees to Chest** – 1 minute

15 **Reclining Twist** – 1 minute then repeat on other side

16 **Banana** – 1 minute then repeat on other side

17 **Shoulder Stand** – 1 minute

18 **Corpse Pose** – 5–10 minutes

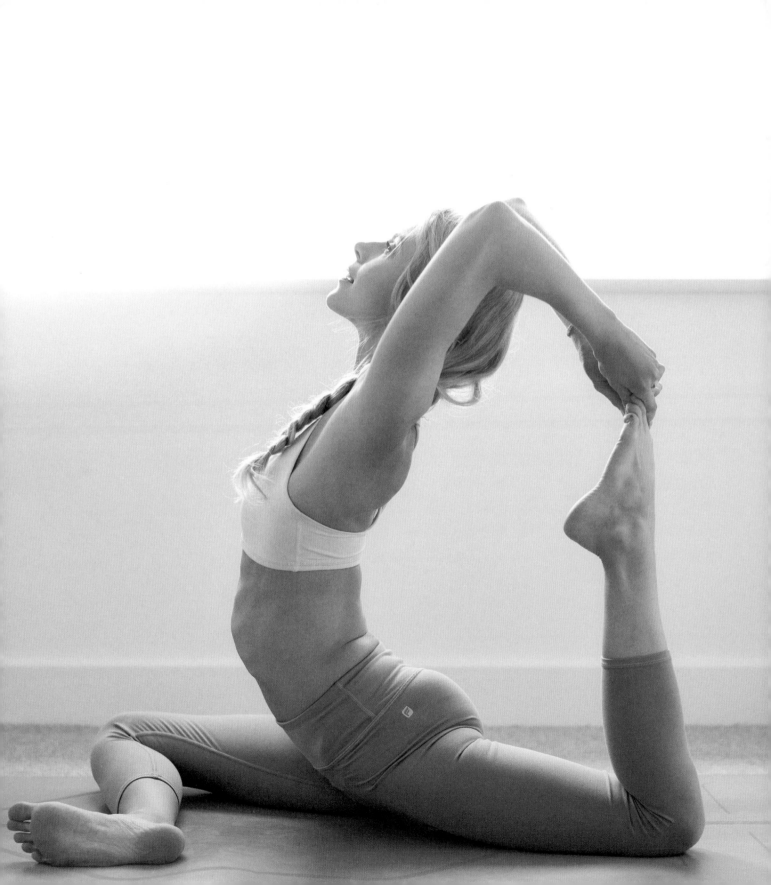

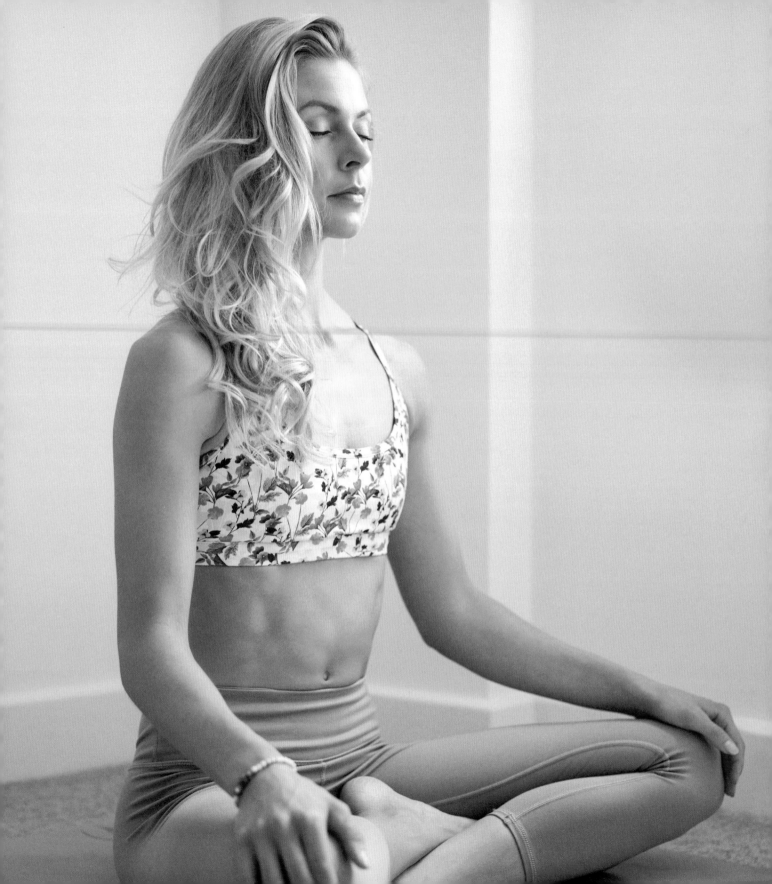

Part 5: Meditations

Guided meditations are a powerful way to elicit transformation in your life. These scripts guide you into a place of relaxation before taking you on a journey to help reduce stress, increase self-compassion, and help you unwind. The beauty of guided meditations like these is that they can bring about amazing physiological and psychological changes in your everyday life. For each of the meditations that follow find a quiet space and get yourself into any comfortable position you can relax in (this can be seated or lying down). Either read the scripts mindfully and slowly or listen to full versions of the guided meditations at www.NicolaJaneHobbs.com.

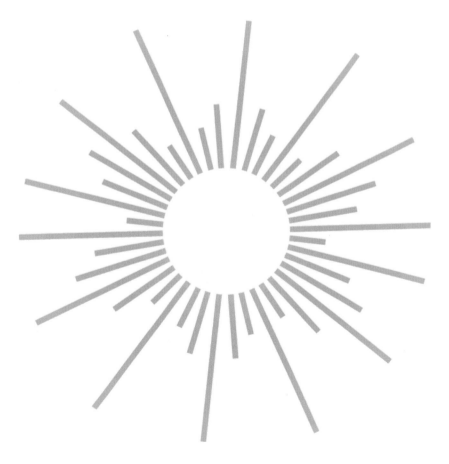

Full Body Relaxation Meditation

Bring your awareness to your breath.

Deepen each inhale and lengthen each exhale.

Now bring your awareness to the top of your head and imagine a peaceful sensation flow down from here, releasing your eye sockets, relaxing your cheeks and your jaw.

Now imagine this feeling flow down through your neck, soothing your shoulders.

Imagine it flow down through your upper arms and into your lower arms, releasing any tension from your upper body out through your fingertips.

Now imagine this feeling of relaxation radiate through your upper back and flow all the way down your spine, releasing and unwinding.

Now bring your awareness to your belly and your chest, feeling it rise and fall with each inhale and each exhale.

Now imagine this peaceful sensation flow through your hips, relaxing the muscles at the front of your thighs and the backs of your thighs.

Imagine it flow down past your knees, soothing your calves, into your feet, taking any tension from anywhere in your body out through the tips of your toes, leaving you feeling relaxed, peaceful and calm.

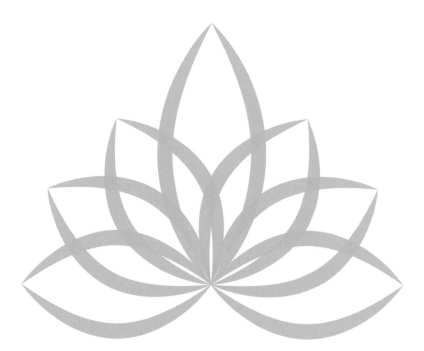

Self-Love Meditation

Bring your awareness to your breath and your body.

Notice how you are feeling in this moment: physically, emotionally, mentally.

Take a deep breath in and as you breathe out allow yourself to fully relax.

Keep your breath relaxed and bring your awareness to any areas where you feel tense or tight and, as you breathe, allow those areas to relax, let that feeling of relaxation radiate throughout your whole body.

Remain relaxed while you meditate calmly and cultivate self-compassion and self-love.

Repeat the following aspirations gently to yourself, inviting love and compassion into your life so that you can thrive:

May I be at peace with myself.

May I allow myself to grow.

May I appreciate who I am.

May I relax.

When I feel down, may I have faith that I will feel happy again.

When I doubt myself, may I find the strength to believe in all that I am.

When I am scared, may I find the courage to follow my heart.

When I fall out of love with myself, may I forgive myself for my mistakes.

When I feel ugly, may I see the beauty in my imperfections.

When my heart feels broken, may I find strength in my vulnerability.

When I don't feel worthy, may I know that I am always good enough.

When I feel insecure, may I accept myself completely.

When I feel lost, may I trust the universe.

May I accept myself.

May I trust myself.

May I nourish myself.

May I love myself.

Bring your awareness back to your breathing. Take a deep breath in and exhale slowly. Notice your feelings of calm, of compassion, of confidence and carry those feelings with you wherever you go.

Stress and Anxiety Relief Meditation

Bring your awareness to your breathing. Deepen the inhale and lengthen the exhale.

Let your shoulders release away from your ears, leaving any thoughts or worries outside of the room and bringing your awareness to the present moment.

Breathe in and breathe out.

Imagine you are in the centre of a storm – a hurricane – there is chaos around you, but you are in the eye of the storm, a place of peace and stillness. Life may be swirling frantically around you but you are safe.

Breathe in and breathe out.

Imagine there is chaos and confusion surrounding you, but you remain safe and calm in the middle of it all.

Breathe in and breathe out.

Imagine this storm is your life. It may be stressful and hectic but you can remain calm and centred as it swirls around outside of you.

Acknowledge that there is a storm in your life, but feel yourself in the eye of it all with a circle of peace surrounding you.

You see the stress and chaos churning around you, but you remain peaceful, relaxed and calm.

Breathe in and breathe out.

You can step into the stress of the storm, you can be dragged into the chaos, or you can remain in the peaceful, tranquil centre of it.

Breathe in and breathe out.

Feel the peace, the calmness, of watching the storm rage around you, but you remain centred, balanced and grounded.

Trusting that everything is OK: calm, soothing, loving.

Breathe in and breathe out.

Feel yourself at peace, grounded here in this moment, knowing that you have a choice as to whether you get sucked into the chaos of the storm, or remain calm and centred in the middle of it.

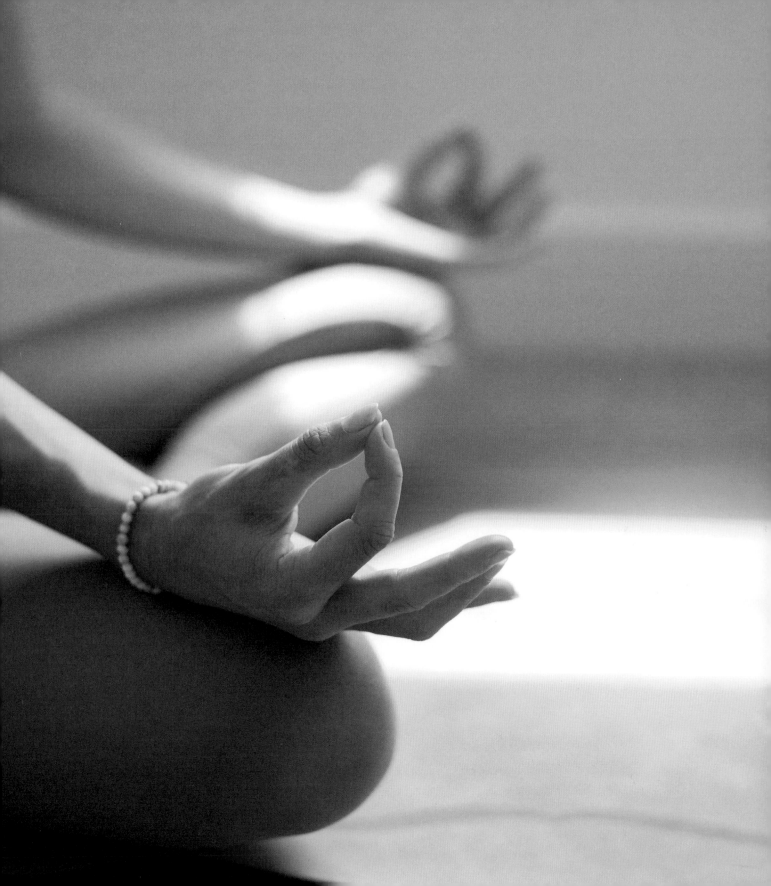

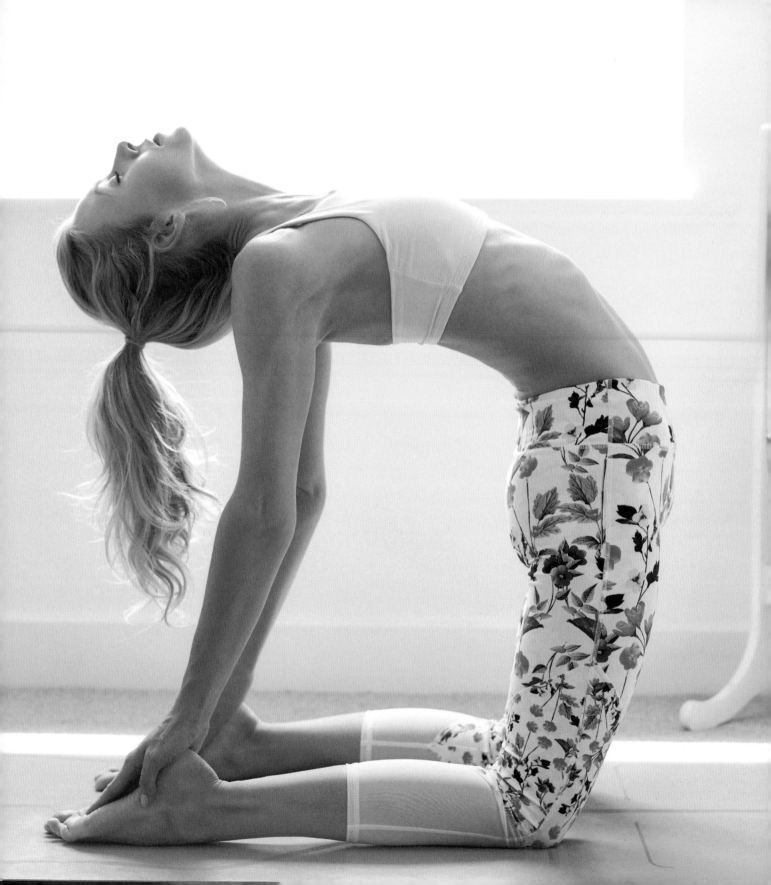

Part 6: Yoga Pose Library

Use the Yoga Pose Library as a guide to help you to get the most out of each pose. Some poses offer modifications so choose a variation that works for you and, as your body begins to respond to your practice by getting stronger and more flexible, explore more challenging variations. It's worth taking some time to explore the poses before you begin the *Thrive Through Yoga* journey so you get a feel of the alignment and intention in each pose and become aware of any areas of resistance or restrictions you can focus on releasing during your journey. Always work with your body rather than against it – just because you can take the full variation of a pose doesn't mean you have to if you are feeling tired, so feel free to pull back whenever you need to.

Baby Bridge

This gentle back bend helps to rebalance the heart, solar plexus and sacral chakras as well as releasing tension from the spine and building strength in the core.

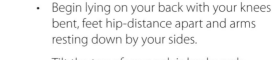

- Begin lying on your back with your knees bent, feet hip-distance apart and arms resting down by your sides.

- Tilt the top of your pelvis backwards to activate your core and lift your hips, pushing your chest towards your chin.

Baby Camel

This pose helps you build strength and find space through your thighs, hips, belly, spine, chest and shoulders.

- Begin kneeling and place your hands on the floor behind you with your fingers facing forward.

- Draw your shoulder blades together, lift your hips and let your head hang back.

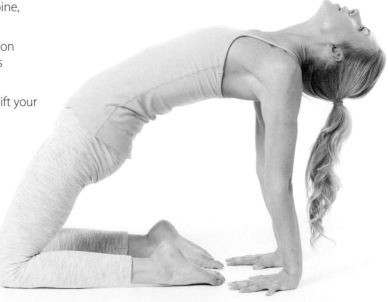

Baby Cobra

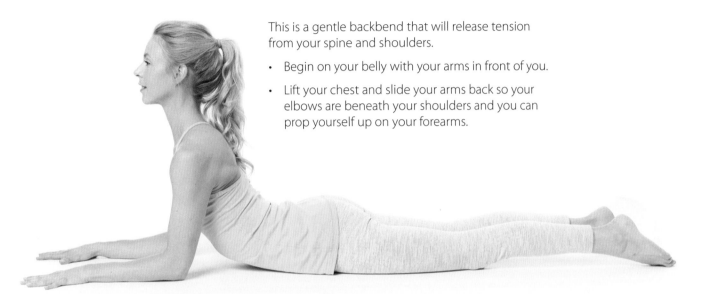

This is a gentle backbend that will release tension from your spine and shoulders.

- Begin on your belly with your arms in front of you.
- Lift your chest and slide your arms back so your elbows are beneath your shoulders and you can prop yourself up on your forearms.

Banana

This is a passive side bend that allows tension to release from the spine, hips and shoulders.

- Begin lying on your back and take hold of your opposite elbow above your head.
- Shift your upper body as far as you can to the side and then shift your feet as far across to the same side as you can. Repeat on the other side.

Bird of Paradise

This is an advanced pose that requires strength, balance and flexibility. Be patient and stay present.

- Begin in Side Angle (see page 170) with your right leg forward and bring your right arm underneath your right leg and left arm behind your back. Interlace your fingers to form a bind.

- Slowly step your left foot next to your right foot. Transition your weight into your left foot and lift your chest, maintaining the bind and bringing your right leg with you. Straighten the right leg and release back down. Repeat on the other side.

Variations: If you can't bind by interlacing your fingers then experiment using a strap by threading it under your leg and taking hold of it with both hands as if your arms are longer.

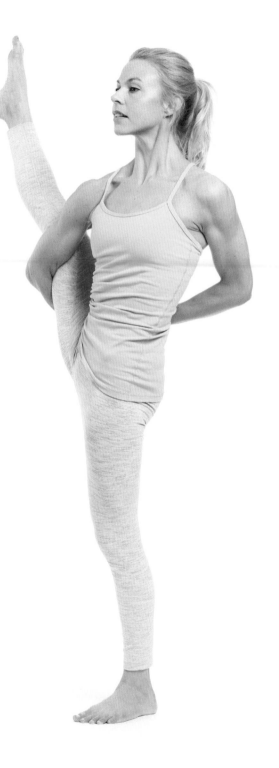

Boat

By focusing on your breath while holding this challenging pose you'll build physical and mental stamina and strength.

- Begin seated with your knees bent and feet flat on the floor. Lean back to lift your feet off the floor and straighten your legs so you are in a V-shape.

- Reach your arms forwards so they are parallel to the floor either side of your legs and look to your toes. Keep your spine long and heart lifted.

Variations: If you find it too challenging to straighten your legs to begin with then keep your legs bent with your toes hovering just above the ground.

Bow

This pose gives you a deep backbend and strong stretch across your chest to help release any stress you're holding in your body.

- Begin lying on your belly, bend your legs and reach back behind you to take hold of your ankles.

- Push your ankles into your palms, draw your shoulder blades together and lift your chest and thighs off the floor to create a bow shape.

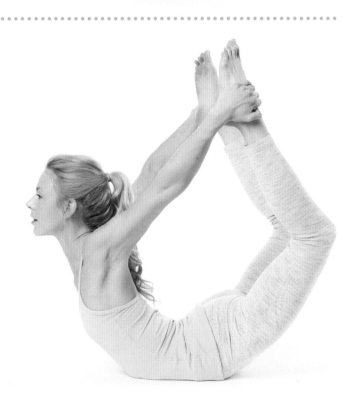

Butterfly

This is a passive forward bend and a hip opener, which helps to draw your awareness inwards, release tension from your pelvis and bring your sacral chakra into balance.

- Begin seated and bring the soles of your feet together with your heels about a foot distance from your groin. Drop your chin to your chest, let your spine round and fold forwards. Gently keep hold of your toes or rest your hands in front of you.

- Focus on relaxing the muscles in your hips and thighs by visualising your knees sinking closer to the floor.

Camel

Backbends increase mobility in the spine as well as stretching out the front of the body to release any blockages from your heart and sacral chakras.

- Begin on your knees with your shoulders stacked over your hips and your hips stacked over your knees and bring your hands to your lower back with your fingers facing down.

- Draw your shoulder blades together and lift your chest as your gently bend backwards to bring your hands to rest on your heels. Keep your hips stacked over your knees and let your head hang back.

Variations: If you feel stiff in your back or have lower back issues then keep your hands on your lower back instead of reaching for your heels.

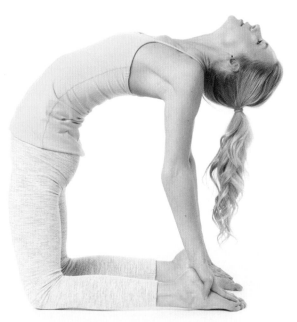

Cat

This is a lovely warm up pose for the spine which also provides a nice massage for your belly organs.

- Begin in Table Top (see page 175). Round your spine, broaden your shoulder blades, tuck your tailbone and drop your head.

Caterpillar

Caterpillar is a relaxing forward bend which soothes the nervous system and eases anxiety.

- Begin seated with your legs out in front of you and your knees soft.
- Drop your chin towards your chest, round your spine and fold forwards slowly. Let your arms rest by the side of your legs. Give your body time and space to open and as it does, release further forwards into the pose.

Variations: If you are really tight down your spine or the backs of your legs it can help to sit on a yoga block.

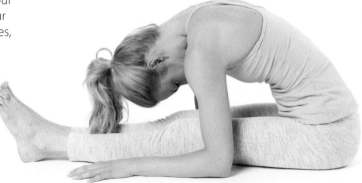

Chair

This pose builds strength in your legs to help you feel centred and grounded.

- Begin in Mountain (see page 159) with your toes, ankles and knees together.
- Bend your knees and drop your hips as you extend your arms overhead.

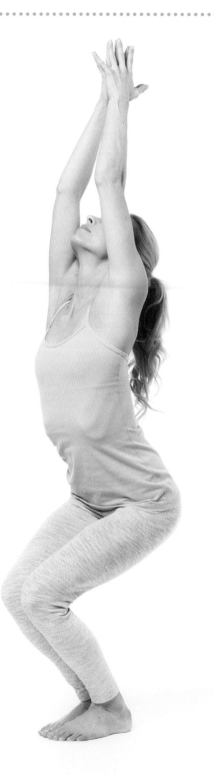

Child's Pose

This is a beautifully restorative pose that releases tension from your spine and calms your mind and nervous system to relieve stress.

- Begin on your hands and knees in Table Top (see page 175) and shift your bottom back towards your heels.

- Either keep your arms out in front of you or bring them back to rest beside you.

Corpse Pose

This is the easiest but also the most difficult pose of them all. In the hectic world we live in, relaxation is greatly undervalued and many of us feel guilty for relaxing. Corpse Pose gives your body and mind the opportunity to relax and fully absorb the benefits of your yoga practice.

- Lie down on your back and begin by taking a deep inhalation, stretching your arms above your head, pointing your toes and squeezing every muscle in your body. As you exhale release all the tension from your body, bring your arms down by your sides with your palms to the sky and allow your feet to wing out just wider than hip distance.

- Release any control over your breathing and allow every muscle in your body to completely relax. Stay here for as long as you want.

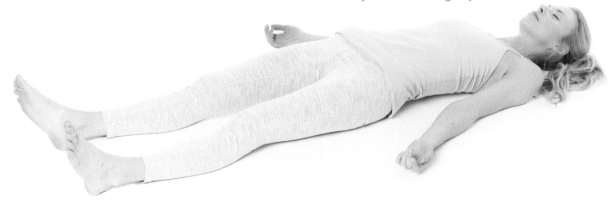

Cow

This is a gentle way to wake up the spine and stretch out the neck.

- Begin in Table Top (see page 175). Curve your back by dropping your belly towards the floor, lifting your heart forwards and lifting your head.

Crocodile

Crocodile is a strengthening pose that teaches you how to balance effort with effortlessness.

- Begin in Plank (see page 161) and bend your elbows into your sides to lower down until you are hovering just above the floor.

- Make sure your hips don't sag or your bottom doesn't lift and keep your neck in line with the rest of your spine by looking down between your thumbs.

Variations: Plank to Crocodile is a challenging transition that you will do every day in the Thrive Sequence. Most people can't do this transition without practice, so build up strength by dropping your knees to the floor before lowering your chest or by lowering all the way down onto your belly.

Crouching Tiger

This pose gives you the feeling of forward momentum – both on the yoga mat and in your life.

- Begin in Down Dog (see page 144) and as you exhale come up on your toes, soften your knees and look between your thumbs.

Crow

This pose requires a combination of strength, balance and focus. Find grounding through your hands to give yourself a stable foundation.

- Begin in a squat and place your hands shoulder-width apart on the floor in front of you.

- Lift your bottom slightly and begin to shift your weight forwards to bring your knees to rest either on the back of your arms or in your armpits.

- Slowly transfer the weight into your hands and point your toes to lift your feet off the ground.

Variations: This is a challenging pose and will take practice. To begin with, leave your toes on the floor and alternate lifting one foot at a time to get a feel for the shape. As you build strength, you'll be able to take both feet off.

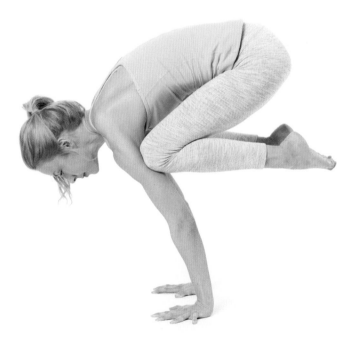

Dancer

This pose combines a balance and a backbend to give you a sense of stability and openness.

- Begin in Mountain (see page 159) and bring your left heel towards your left buttock. Reach back with your left hand to take hold of the inside of your left foot and extend your right arm to the sky.

- On an exhale lean forward as you kick your left foot into your left hand to create an arch in your spine. Breathe. Repeat on the other side.

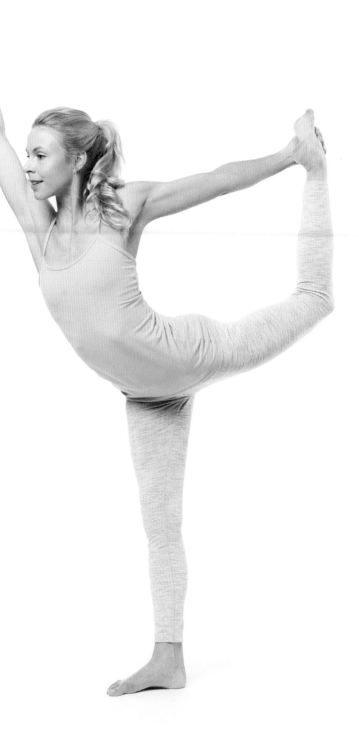

Deer

Deer pose is a gentle but deep hip opener which brings the body into balance through internal and external rotation of your hips.

- Begin seated with the soles of your feet together in Butterfly (see page 136). Swing your right leg around behind you and position the right foot so your right knee is at a right angle. Move your left foot forwards until your thigh and shin make a right angle.

- Focus on releasing both buttocks to the ground and as your hips relax, move your right foot further away from your right hip.

- To exit the pose, lift both knees to the sky, and then repeat on the other side.

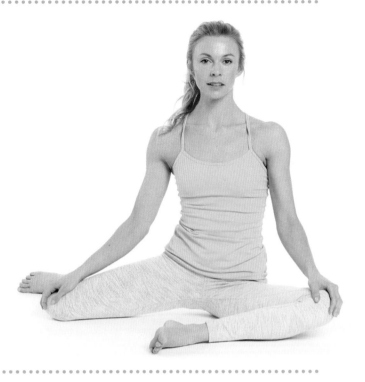

Dolphin

By strengthening your shoulders and stretching your chest Dolphin helps to rebalance the heart chakra and increase self-acceptance and self-compassion.

- Begin in Table Top (see page 175) and bring your forearms to the floor.

- Hook your toes and lift your bottom to the sky as you would for Down Dog. Focus on pushing your chest back towards your thighs and lifting your shoulders up and away from your wrists.

Variations: If your shoulders are tight, instead of having your forearms parallel on the floor interlace your fingers. If your hamstrings feel tight, lift your heels and bend your knees slightly so you can push your chest back.

Dolphin Plank

This Plank variation will activate your core and help to rebalance your solar plexus chakra to ignite passion and purpose.

- Begin in Dolphin pose (see page 143) and shift your shoulders forwards until they are stacked over your elbows at the same time as walking your feet back until your spine is parallel to the floor.

- Squeeze your bottom, brace your belly and tuck in your tailbone slightly.

Down Dog

Down Dog epitomises the balance between strength and flexibility by building strength and openness in your shoulders, spine and legs.

- Begin in Table Top (see page 175) with your shoulders stacked over your wrists.

- Hook your toes under, straighten your legs and lift your bottom to the sky so you are in an upturned V-shape.

- Keep pushing your chest back towards your thighs and releasing your heels towards the floor.

Dragon Flying High

This is a passive version of a lunge. It releases stress from your hips gently and passively.

- Begin in Table Top (see page 175) and step your right foot between your hands. Slide your left knee back as far as you can while keeping your right knee stacked over your right ankle.

- Lift your chest and rest your hands on your knee. Allow gravity to help you release deeper into the pose. Repeat on the other leg.

Notes: If you feel pressure in your back knee then place a cushion under it to give it some padding. As your hips open you'll find you begin to rest on top of the thigh which will take any pressure off the kneecap.

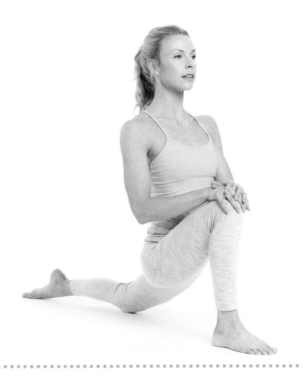

Dragon Flying Low

This pose is a deep hip opener which helps to rebalance the sacral chakra and release any emotions you have been holding on to.

- Begin in Table Top (see page 175) and step your right foot to the outside of your right hand. Slide your left knee back as far as you can while keeping your right knee stacked over your right ankle.

- Either stay on your hands or make your way down onto your forearms. Hold this pose passively and focus on relaxing into it. Repeat on your left leg.

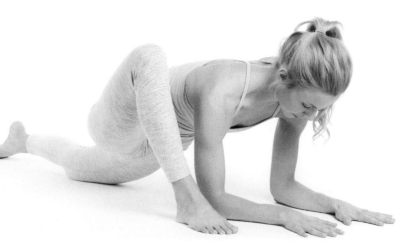

Eagle

Eagle draws energy inwards to help you focus on your balance and give you strength and stability for the pose.

- Begin in Mountain (see page 159). Cross your right arm over your left, bending your elbows so your forearms are vertical, and then bring your palms together. Next, bend your knees and cross your left leg over your right, squeeze your thighs together and hook the toes of your left foot behind your right calf.

- Drop your hips, lift your elbows and wrap your shoulder blades around the back of your ribcage to stretch your upper back. Breathe and soften into the pose for a few breaths.

- Repeat on the opposite side.

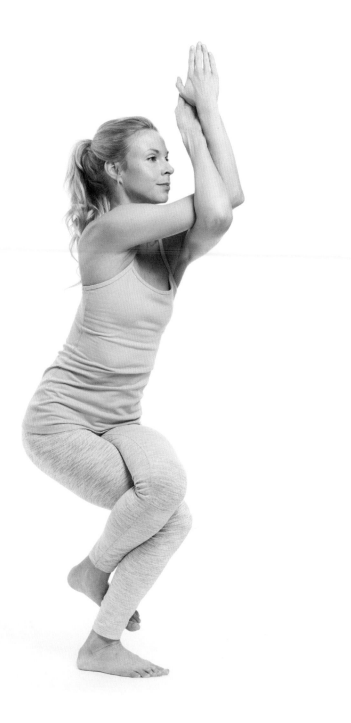

Easy Pose

This is a simple comfortable position that allows you to focus on your breath, set your intention and meditate.

- Sit on the floor cross legged, with your spine long and your shoulders relaxed.

Variations: If you don't find this comfortable then sit with a yoga block or a couple of cushions underneath your bottom to help tilt your pelvis.

Notes: Switch which way you cross your legs each time you sit in the pose to keep your body in balance.

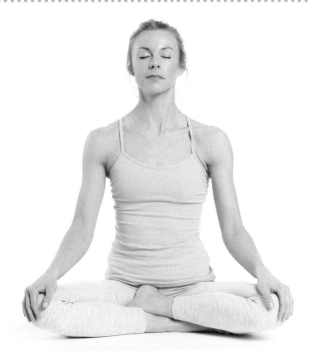

Egg Stand

Getting upside down challenges us to get outside of our comfort zone, but we need to do it slowly and steadily to find confidence in ourselves. Egg Stand is a gentle way for you to find balance while upside down.

- Begin on your hands and knees and bend your arms to lower your head to the floor about 50cm (20 inches) in front of your hands so you are creating a triangle with your head as the top point.

- Straighten your legs and shift your weight into your hands and head. Walk your toes towards your hands until your bottom is stacked over your hips.

- Step your right knee onto your right upper arm and your left knee onto your left upper arm, hugging your heels into your bottom.

Variations: If you're afraid of falling then begin practising with your back against a wall and slowly work your way away from it.

Notes: If you have any neck issues then avoid this pose.

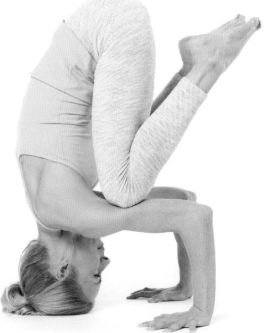

Forward Bend Balance

Balancing on different areas of our body helps teach us how to ground ourselves when we find ourselves in challenging situations in life.

- Begin seated, bend your knees and take hold of your ankles, heels or big toes.

- Shift your weight back slightly to lift your feet off the ground. Keep your knees together and slowly straighten your legs as you lean backwards to counterbalance your legs.

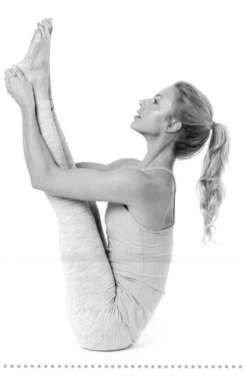

Four Face Breath

This is a simple technique you can use in times of stress or anxiety to help you let go of any worries and bring your awareness to the present moment.

- Begin in Easy Pose (see page 147). Rest your eyes and take a deep inhalation.

- As you exhale look to your right.

- Inhale and bring your head back to centre.

- Exhale and look to the left.

- Inhale back to centre.

- Exhale and let your head fall back so you feel a stretch in the front of your neck.

- Inhale back to centre.

- Exhale and look down.

- Inhale back to centre and repeat the sequence.

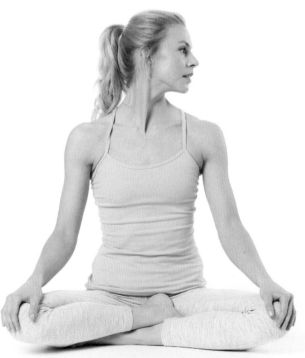

Goddess

This pose strengthens your core and thighs as well as stretching your inner thighs and releasing tension from your hips.

- Begin in a wide legged position with your hips facing the long edge of your mat.

- Bend your knees and drop your hips until your thighs are parallel to the floor and bring your palms to your heart.

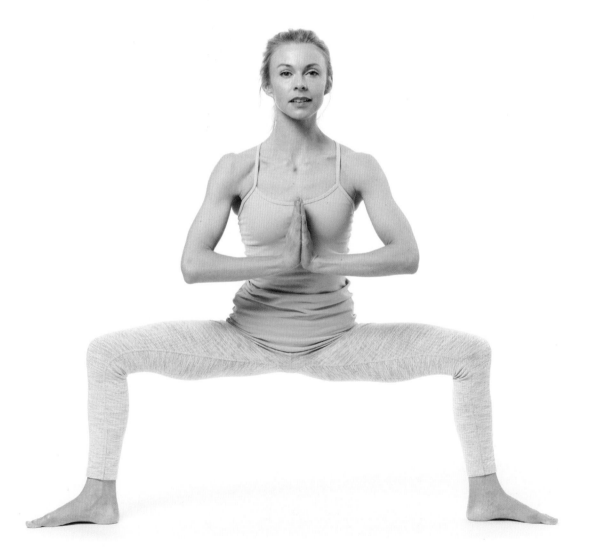

Half Moon

By bending sideways in this pose you release tension from your spine, by stretching upwards you create a sense of lift and openness, and by keeping your chest open to the sky you release blockages from your heart chakra.

- Begin in Upward Salute (see page 180), and on an exhale lean to your right to create an even side bend through your spine.

- Return to Upward Salute and repeat to the left.

Half Moon Balance

This is a challenging balance and hip opener. Focus on rooting to the ground through your standing leg so you can create stability and find more space in your hips.

- Begin in Warrior 2 (see page 181) with your right leg forward, and place your right hand on the floor about a foot in front of your right toes. Rest your left fingertips on the floor next to your right foot to help you keep your balance.

- Keep your hips facing the long edge of the mat and slowly straighten your right leg as you lift your left leg until it is parallel to the floor. Reach your left hand to the sky. Repeat on the left leg.

Variations: If it feels as though the arm on the floor is too short then place a block under your hand to give you more height.

Half Splits

By stretching out the back of your legs this pose is great preparation for full splits. It helps teach you that baby steps are an important part of your journey.

- Begin in Dragon Flying High (see page 145) with one foot forward. Bring your hands to the floor either side of your foot.

- Shift your hips back until they are stacked above your back knee and your front leg is straight. Flex the front foot and fold forwards. Repeat on the other leg.

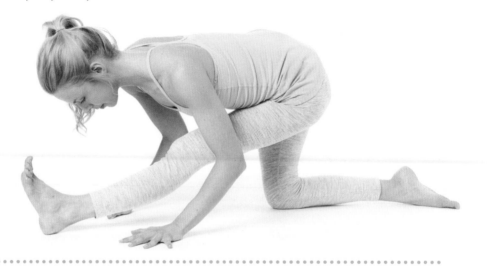

Happy Baby

Happy Baby is a pose you often see newborns embracing. It is a deep hip opener and also stretches the hamstrings and decompresses the lower back, to leave you feeling calm and refreshed.

- Lie down on your back in Knees to Chest pose (see page 155) and take hold of the soles of your feet. Bring your shins so they are vertical to the floor and the soles of your feet are facing the ceiling.

- With your feet aligned above your knees, engage your biceps to pull your knees towards your armpits. Keep your head and shoulders relaxed on the floor.

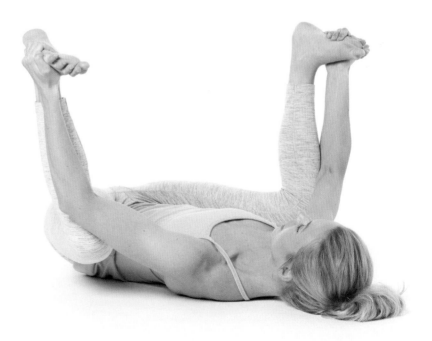

Headstand

Headstands are a wonderful way to improve overall wellbeing by stimulating the hypothalamus and pituitary glands, helping to decongest the lymph glands and stimulate circulation.

- Begin in Egg Stand (see page 147) and slowly lift your knees off your upper arms and bring them together to form a tuck shape.

- Straighten your legs towards the sky, keeping your weight spread evenly between your hands and your head.

Variations: If you're afraid of falling then begin practising with your back against a wall and slowly work your way away from it.

Notes: *If you have any neck issues then avoid this pose.*

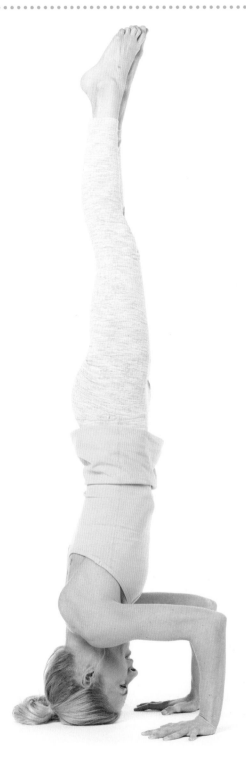

Head to Knee Pose

This forward bend helps to calm anxiety while releasing tension from the back of your legs.

- Start in Mountain pose (see page 159) and take a step about a metre back with your left foot. Turn the toes of your left foot out slightly to help you find balance.

- Bring your hands to your hips, and on an exhale fold forwards to bring your chest towards your right thigh. Release your fingers to rest on your shin, ankle or the floor. Lengthen your spine with each inhale and fold deeper with each exhale. Repeat on the other leg.

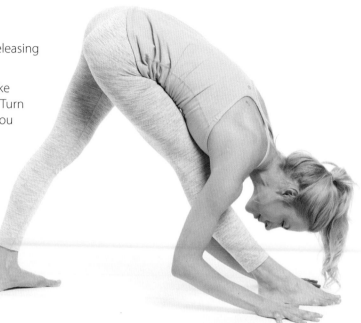

Humble Warrior

This adds a backbend and a forward bend into a traditional Warrior pose to challenge your focus and help you grow stronger.

- Begin in Warrior 1 (see page 181) with one foot forward, and lift your back heel. Interlace your fingers behind your back and draw your shoulder blades together to open your chest.

- Fold forward to rest your chest on your front thigh and bring your arms up and over your head, looking towards your big toe. Repeat on the other leg.

Knees to Chest Pose

This is a calming and restorative pose which takes pressure off the lower back and allows your nervous system to relax.

- Begin on your back and hug your knees into your chest. Wrap your arms around your legs, keeping your belly, shoulders and back relaxed.

- Rock from side to side to massage out your spine.

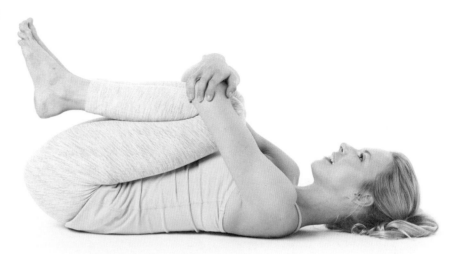

Legs Up the Wall

This is a restorative pose that brings your feet above your heart to help you relax and restore. If you have trouble sleeping then this is a good pose to practise before bed.

- Sit sideways against the wall and swing your legs around so you are lying on your back with your legs up the wall. Bring your bottom as close to the wall as you can and straighten your legs, resting your heels on the wall.

- Spread your arms out sideways. Rest here for as long as you need to.

Lift and Lengthen

By keeping our chest lifted even as we're folding forwards we learn to keep our heart open.

- Begin in a Standing Forward Bend (see page 173) with your hands resting on your shins, ankles or the floor.

- As you inhale lift halfway up so your spine is parallel to the floor. Draw your shoulders away from your ears and lift your heart forwards to create length in your spine.

- As you exhale fold forwards into the space you've created.

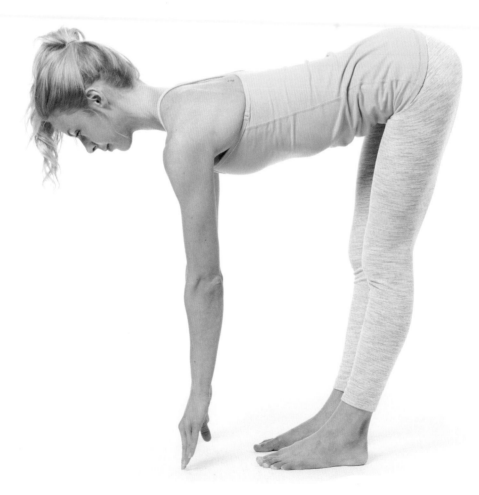

Locust

By stabilising your lower back this pose helps to create both strength and openness.

- Begin lying on your belly with your arms by your side.

- Push your pubic bone towards the mat, draw your shoulder blades together and lift your chest and legs off the floor.

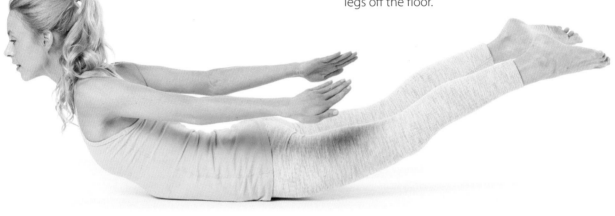

Low Boat

This pose builds strength in the core and helps to stabilise the spine to give you stability and confidence in more challenging poses like Headstand.

- Begin lying on your back with your legs straight out on the floor and your arms by your side.

- Push your lower back towards the floor, draw your belly button towards your spine and lift your shoulders and feet about 20 cm (8 inches) off the floor.

Variations: If you have any back issues, place your hands under your bottom with your palms facing down. To make the pose more challenging reach your arms overhead.

Low Lunge

This pose helps create space in your hips, spine, shoulders and chest.

- Begin in Down Dog (see page 144) and step one foot between your hands. Drop your back knee to the mat and lift your fingers to the sky. Drop your hips to find stability as you reach upwards to create openness. Repeat on the other leg.

Melting Heart

This passive backbend is a beautiful way to release any hurt from your heart and create space for love and peace.

- Begin in Table Top (see page 175) and walk your fingers forwards as you release your chest down towards the floor.

- Rest your forehead on the floor and keep your bottom stacked over your hips as you relax through your shoulders and allow your chest to sink closer to the floor.

Mountain

This is a beautiful way to ground yourself and tune into your body in between poses.

- Stand with your toes, ankles, and knees together and heart lifted.

- Bring your palms together in front of your heart and let your shoulders relax away from your ears.

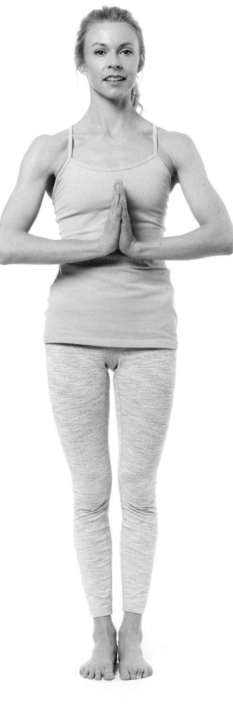

Ocean Breath

This is a balancing and calming breath which increases oxygenation and builds internal heat in the body.

- Sit comfortably with your spine upright and take a couple of long deep breaths.

- Inhale through your nose, and exhale through your mouth. With each exhalation make a 'hhhaaaaa' sound as if you are trying to steam up a mirror.

- Now continue to make the same sound as you exhale but close your mouth so you are constricting the back of your throat to make a soft ocean sound.

Pendant

This is a strong arm balance and core pose which will give you a challenge to work towards and a huge sense of accomplishment when you get there.

- Begin in Table Top (see page 175).

- Sit back to bring your bottom towards your heels and slide your hands back so they are positioned mid-thigh. Round your spine, push the floor away through your hands and hug your knees up into your chest, bringing your heels with you.

Variations: This is a challenging pose but you can get the same benefits by leaving your toes on the ground and just drawing your knees into your chest. You can also place blocks under your hands to make it easier to lift yourself.

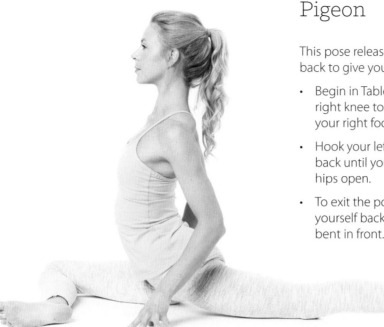

Pigeon

This pose releases tension from the hips and lower back to give you a sense of openness and release.

- Begin in Table Top (see page 175) and bring your right knee to the outside of your right wrist and your right foot towards your left wrist.

- Hook your left toes under and lift your left knee back until you find your edge and feel your hips open.

- To exit the pose, hook your left toes under and lift yourself back to Table Top. Repeat with the left leg bent in front.

Plank

This pose is a great way to build physical and psychological strength.

- Begin in Table Top (see page 175) with your shoulders stacked over your wrists and step your feet back so your legs are straight.

- Squeeze your buttocks, brace your belly and push the floor away through your hands.

Variations: If you experience any back pain or feel the full pose is too strong to begin with then drop your knees to the floor or raise your hands on a low surface making sure you keep your core muscles engaged.

Notes: When practising Plank in the Thrive Sequence you will step or jump back from a Standing Forward Bend instead of pushing up from Table Top.

Plough

This is a beautiful pose to calm the brain and relieve stress and fatigue.

- Begin lying on your back and roll your legs up and overhead, supporting your lower back with your hands. Either keep your legs parallel to the floor or bring your toes to the floor behind your head.

- Once you feel stable, release your hands from your lower back, interlace your fingers and push your hands towards the floor.

Ragdoll

Like the name suggests, this is a passive pose that encourages you to dangle in a forward bend to release control and calm your nervous system.

- Begin in Mountain (see page 159) with your feet about hip distance apart.

- Soften your knees and fold forwards, letting your spine round and your head hang. Take hold of your opposite elbow and dangle here passively, swaying gently from side to side.

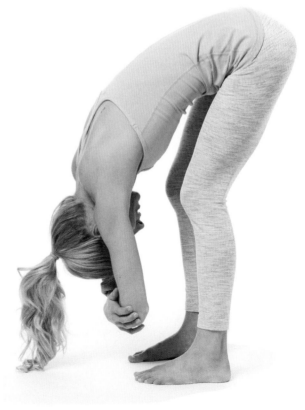

Reclining Twist

Passive twists are perfect for twisting out any tension from the spine and allowing your body to fully relax and release.

- Begin lying on your back and hug your right knee into your chest. Take hold of the outside of your right knee with your left hand and bring your right leg across your body. Keep both shoulder blades on the floor and look over your right shoulder.

- Either keep your right leg bent or see if you can straighten it and take hold of your right foot with your left forefingers to increase the twist.

- Come out of the pose by releasing your foot, rolling onto your back and hugging your knees into your chest before repeating with your left leg.

Reverse Table Top

This pose builds full body strength to give you confidence in yourself, and releases tension from your chest to open your heart chakra.

- Begin seated with your legs bent in front of you and the soles of your feet on the floor. Reach your hands back behind you with your fingertips facing forwards.

- Straighten your arms and draw your shoulder blades together to open the chest. Squeeze your bottom, lift your hips and let your head hang back.

Reverse Warrior

Reverse Warrior is great for stretching and strengthening the body. The pose builds strength in the front thigh while opening the chest and stretching the entire upper body, which will lengthen the spine and leave you feeling confident and determined.

- Begin in Warrior 2 (see page 181) with your right leg bent and lean back to bring your left hand down towards your left knee and reach your right arm up and over with your palm facing the floor behind you.

- To help keep your chest open, you can half bind your left arm behind your back to take hold of the top of your right thigh.

- Repeat on the left leg.

Seated Forward Bend

This is a beautiful pose to calm your nervous system and help ease anxiety.

- Begin in Staff Pose (see page 173) and as you inhale reach your fingertips to the sky.

- As you exhale fold forwards by hinging from your hips and taking hold of your shins, ankles or toes.

- Lengthen your heart forwards as you inhale and fold deeper as you exhale.

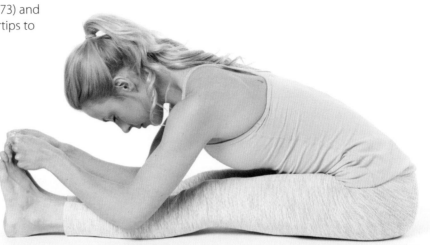

Seated Shoulder Stretch

This is a beautiful heart opener and stretches out your chest and down your arms to create balance with the strengthening poses.

- Begin seated with your legs bent in front of you and the soles of your feet on the floor. Reach your hands back behind you as far as you can with your fingertips facing forwards.

- Step your feet forward, lift your bottom and bring it towards your heels until you feel a stretch in your shoulders then lower your bottom to the ground. Bend your arms a little and squeeze your elbows towards each other.

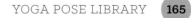

Seated Side Bend

By bending sideways you release tension from your spine which will help you to relieve stress and calm your nervous system.

- Begin seated in Easy Pose (see page 147) and as you inhale reach both hands to the sky.

- As you exhale lean over to one side, placing your hand to the floor and reaching your other arm up and over.

- Repeat on the other side.

Seated Twist

This gentle twist is a great way to release stress from your spine and stimulate your internal organs.

- Begin seated in Easy Pose (see page 147) and as you inhale reach both hands to the sky.

- As you exhale, begin twisting to your left to bring your right hand to your left knee and release your left hand down behind you. Lengthen your spine with each inhale and twist a bit more as you exhale. Repeat on the other side.

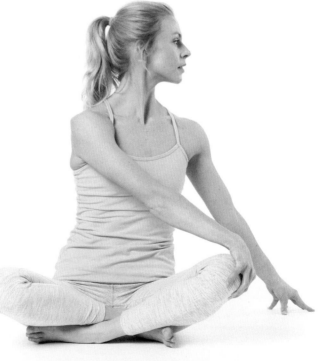

Shaking the Tree

Our body, just like other mammals', shakes naturally after trauma to release tension. These are known as neurogenic tremors, and it is the body's natural way to release stress. Shaking the Tree taps into this inbuilt mechanism by encouraging you to shake to help you release stress and tension from your body so you sleep better, move better and feel better.

- Begin in Mountain with your feet hip distance apart. Close your eyes and gently begin bouncing up and down, shaking your arms and allowing your body to move freely.

Shoelace

Shoelace is a deep hip opener and a psychologically challenging pose to remain in. It teaches you that even when it feels like life is tying you in knots, you can choose to relax and find release.

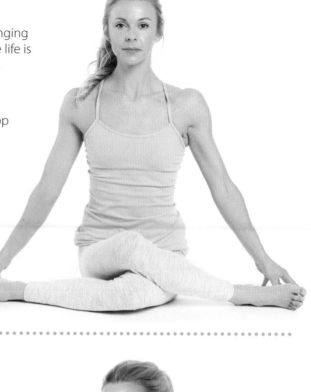

- Begin sitting cross legged on the floor and slide your left foot under your right leg to bring your left heel to the outside of your right buttock. Stack your right knee on top of your left knee and bring your right heel to the outside of your left buttock.

- Anchor your buttocks to the floor and then bring both feet as far forward away from your buttocks as you can while keeping your knees stacked.

- Focus on relaxing your hips and then repeat on the other side.

Variations: If you have any knee issues then stay in Half Shoelace with the bottom leg straight.

Shoulder Squeezing Pose

This is a challenging pose that will ignite your core and help you find balance on your hands.

- Squat down with your feet about shoulder width apart and then tilt your chest forwards and lift your hips so that your thighs are parallel to the floor.

- Reach your right arm between your legs and place your right hand on the floor to the outside of your right foot, getting your right shoulder as far under your right thigh as you can. Repeat with the left arm.

- Press your hands into the floor and slowly rock back to transfer the weight from your feet to your hands. Squeeze your inner thighs into your arms, lift your feet and cross your ankles.

Shoulder Stand

Shoulder Stand is a strengthening inversion which helps to calm your nervous system, balance your hormones and stimulate your throat chakra which can help with self-expression.

- Begin in Plough pose and bring your hands to your lower back.

- Slowly lift your toes towards the ceiling until your legs are vertical.

Variations: Avoid Shoulder Stand if you have neck issues and practise Legs Up the Wall pose instead.

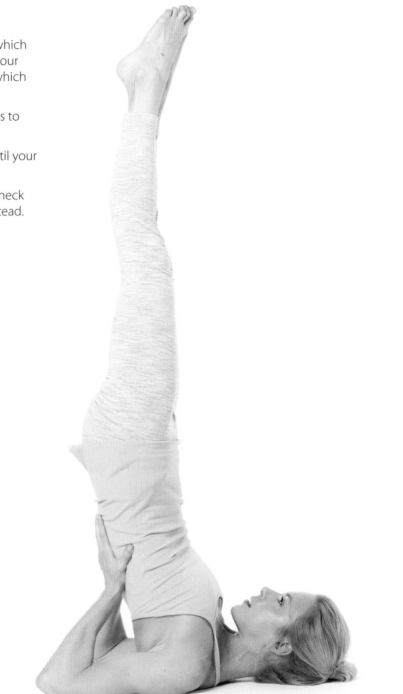

Side Angle

This pose strengthens your legs while opening your chest, to allow you to focus on the power of your breath.

- Begin in Warrior 2 (page 181) with your right leg bent and bring your right fingertips to rest on the floor on the inside of your right foot. Shoot your left arm overhead as if you are throwing a spear so you create a diagonal line of energy from the outside of your left foot through your left fingertips. Focus on rotating your chest open to the sky.

- Repeat on your left leg.

Variations: If your inner thighs feel tight and you find it difficult to reach the floor then rest your forearm on your thigh instead. If you want to deepen the pose: with your right leg forwards, wrap your right arm under your right thigh and your left arm behind your back and interlace your fingers to form a bind.

Screaming Pigeon

This provides a strong stretch to your thighs and creates openness in your hips to release any blockages in your sacral chakra.

- Begin in Pigeon (see page 161) and bend your left leg and reach back with your left hand to bring your left heel towards your left buttock. Repeat on the other side.

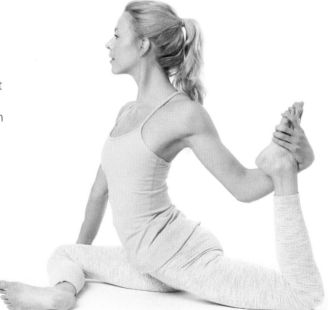

Sleeping Butterfly

This is a lovely restorative pose that allows your whole body to relax and rebalance.

- Begin lying on your back with your knees bent and your heels about a foot away from your bottom.

- Let your knees fall out to the side and bring the soles of your feet together.

- Rest your hands on your belly and focus on it rising as you inhale and falling as you exhale.

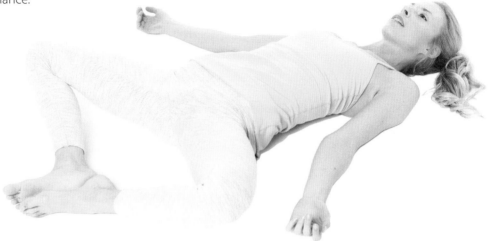

Sleeping Pigeon

This is a beautiful pose to get to know your body and notice where you hold stress.

- Begin in Pigeon (see page 161) and fold forwards by lying your chest on your shin and either resting your forearms or your forehead on the ground in front of you.

- Relax here and then when you're ready to exit, lift your chest back to Pigeon and repeat on the other side.

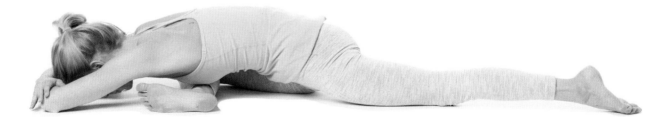

Splits

Splits are a wonderful way to understand how growth and transformation take time. The splits require practice and patience and can often take months or years to release all the way down.

- Begin in Half Splits (see page 152) and slowly slide the front foot forwards until you find your edge. Stay here for a few breaths to allow your hips to relax and see if you can release a bit deeper as your body opens. Repeat on the other side.

Notes: Work slowly and gently in this pose. Instead of forcing yourself into it allow your body to release and find space.

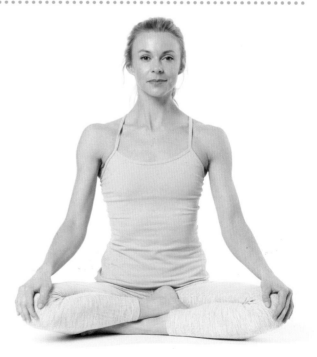

Square Breathing

This is a calming breathing technique that works beautifully to relieve stress and anxiety. It redirects your focus away from any stresses of the external world to your inner stillness.

- Sit comfortably with your spine upright and take a couple of long deep breaths.

- Inhale for a count of four, hold your breath for a count of four, exhale for a count of four, and hold the exhalation for a count of four. This is one cycle of Square Breathing.

Staff Pose

This is a seated version of Mountain and is great to practise in between other poses to bring your body back into balance and tune into any changes you feel in your body or mind.

- Begin seated and lengthen your legs straight out in front of you. Place your hands either side of you with your fingertips facing sideways and lengthen the crown of your head to the sky.

Standing Forward Bend

Forward bends are a lovely way to ease anxiety and calm mental chatter.

- Begin with your feet hip-distance apart and bring your hands to your hips.

- As you inhale lengthen your spine and as you exhale fold forwards by hinging from your hips.

- Release your fingers down to take hold of your shins, ankles, toes or to rest on the floor.

- With each inhale lift and lengthen, and as you exhale see if you can fold deeper into the pose.

Notes: *When practising a forward bend in the Thrive Sequence, dive straight into it from Upward Salute instead of bringing your hands to your hips.*

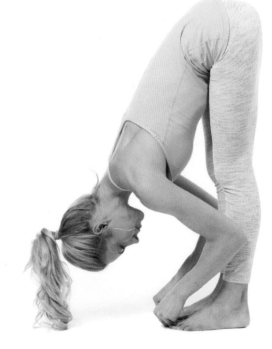

Stomach Pumping Breath

This is an energising breathing technique which refreshes your body and mind.

- Begin in Easy Pose (see page 147) and take a couple of full deep breaths.

- Exhale forcefully through your nose in rapid succession 10 times, snapping your belly in at a rate of one exhalation per second. The force of the exhale should create enough suction for the inhale to be automatic.

- On the tenth exhale, inhale and exhale deeply and return to your normal breath for 10–15 seconds before repeating.

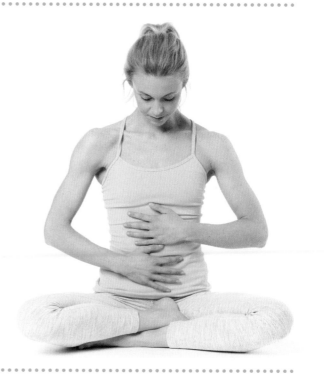

Straddle

We tend to hold a lot of tension in our hips so Straddle is a lovely pose to release any tightness. Sometimes you can feel an emotional release after you release physical tension from your hips so be gentle with yourself after practising hip openers.

- Begin seated and spread your legs wide. Allow your spine to round and fold forwards by walking your fingertips forwards.

- Relax here and play your edge by creeping your fingers further forwards as your body opens.

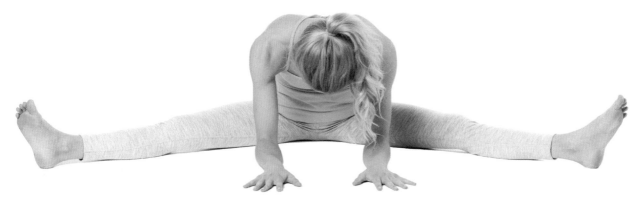

Straddle Balance

As well as balancing on our feet, it is helpful to be able to balance on other areas of our body. This pose challenges you to find balance on your bottom using strength in your core and length in your spine.

- Begin seated, bend your knees and take hold of your big toes. Lean back, lift your feet off the floor and slowly straighten your legs into a wide legged position.

- Keep your chest lifted and core activated to help your balance.

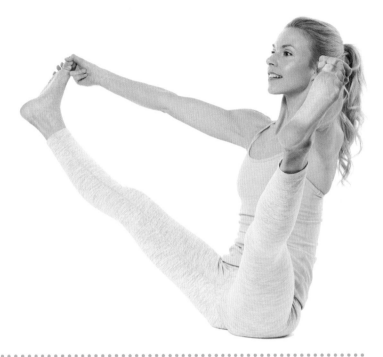

Table Top

This is a great pose to practise grounding and alignment in.

- Come onto your hands and knees and bring your shoulders over your hands and your hips over your knees.

- Keep your neck in line with the rest of your spine by looking between your thumbs.

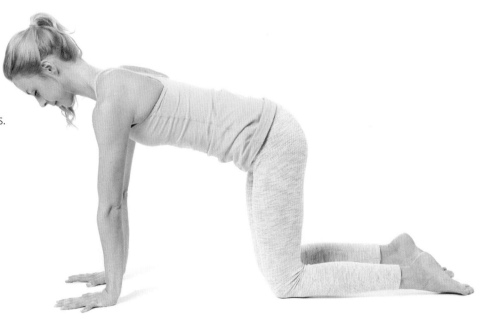

Three Legged Dog

By lifting one leg we are learning how to find balance even when life feels a little askew.

- Begin in Down Dog (see page 144) and as you inhale lift your right leg to the sky making sure you keep your hips even.

- Keep the right leg straight and keep pushing your chest back towards your left thigh. Repeat on the other side.

Tiger

Tiger is a beautiful backbend which releases tension from your spine and builds strength through your core.

- Begin in Table Top (see page 175) and reach your right foot to the sky with the leg bent. Reach back with your left arm to take hold of your right ankle and push your right foot into your left hand to create lift. Repeat on the other side.

Tree

Tree Pose teaches you to root yourself to the ground to help you feel centred and balanced.

- Begin in Mountain (see page 159) and bring your left foot up to rest on your right inner thigh.

- Bring your palms to your heart and find something static in front of you to focus on to help you balance. Repeat on the other side.

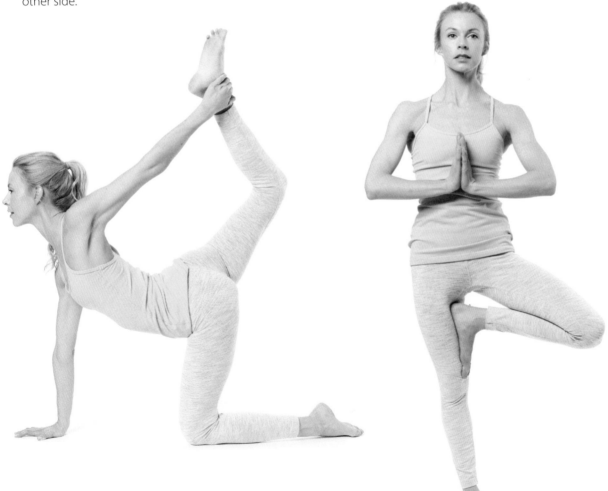

Triangle

This is a great full-body stretch that helps to bring your awareness to any muscles that are feeling particularly tight.

- Begin in Warrior 2 (see page 181) with your right leg forward. Straighten your right leg and reach over, hinging from your hips, before bringing your right hand down to rest against your inner shin or ankle and extending your left arm to the sky.

- Stretch from fingertip to fingertip with each inhale, and with each exhale rotate your chest open to the sky. Repeat on the left leg.

Twisted Side Angle

This pose works your lower body and your core to produce a detoxifying twist.

- Begin in Mountain (see page 159) and step your left foot back about 1.5 metres. Drop your left knee to the floor and bring your palms to your heart.

- Rotate over your right leg from your core to bring your left elbow to the outside of your right knee so your right elbow is facing the sky.

- Lift your left knee off the floor and straighten the leg. Repeat on the other side.

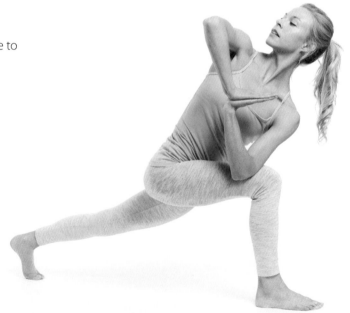

Twisted Triangle

The challenging twist of this pose develops a sense of balance and grounding from which you can stretch and extend.

- Begin in Head to Knee pose (see page 154) with your right foot forward. Push your left hand into the floor on the little toe side of your right foot and as you inhale reach your right hand to the sky.

- Repeat on the left side.

Variations: To make the pose slightly easier, with your right foot forward place your left hand on the inside of your right foot instead of the outside.

Up Dog

This is a beautiful back bend that will release tension from your chest and open your heart.

- Begin lying on your belly and slide your hands back so they are either side of your chest.

- As you inhale straighten your arms and lift your chest. Draw your shoulder blades together and lift your heart forwards. You can leave your knees on the floor or push the tops of your feet into the floor to lift your kneecaps for a more challenging pose.

Variations: If you have any back issues or feel very stiff then start with Baby Cobra (see page 133) and build up to Up Dog as your body starts to open.

Upward Salute

This poses gives us a sense of rooting and rising –
grounding ourselves while also growing.

- Begin in Mountain (see page 159) and as you
  inhale reach your arms above your head, bringing
  your palms together.

- Let your shoulders relax away from your ears and
  look towards your thumbs.

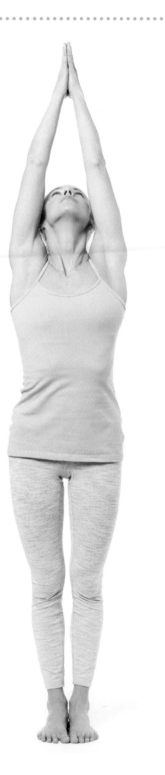

Warrior 1

Warrior 1 teaches us that there is no war within us – we are on our own side.

- Begin in Mountain (see page 159) and take a big step back with your left leg. Keep the toes of your right foot facing forwards and turn your left foot out by 45 degrees, or stay on the ball of the foot so you can keep both hips in line.

- Bend your right leg until your front thigh is parallel to the floor and reach your hands to the sky, bringing your palms together.

- Repeat with the left leg forwards.

Notes: In the Thrive Sequence you will enter Warrior 1 through Three Legged Dog by lifting your arms to the sky from Warrior Prep.

Warrior 2

The stability and strength of Warrior 2 embodies the spirit of a Warrior – battling weakness and building inner strength.

- Begin in Mountain pose (see page 159) and take a big step back with your left leg. Keep the toes of your right foot facing forward, turn your left foot out by 45 degrees and open your hips so they are facing the long edge of your mat.

- Bend your right knee until your thigh is parallel to the floor and spread your arms out wide.

- Repeat on the left leg.

Notes: In the Thrive Sequence you will enter Warrior 2 through Warrior 1 by opening your hips and spreading your arms wide.

Warrior 3

This is a strong balance which will give you a sense of strength and grounding as you launch forwards into the next stage of your journey.

- Begin in Warrior 1 (see page 181) with your right leg forward and palms to your heart and lift your back heel.

- Push your weight onto your front foot as you launch forwards, lift your back leg and straighten your front leg so your chest and back leg are parallel to the floor. Repeat on the left leg.

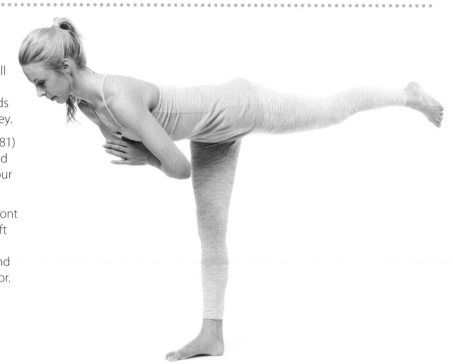

Warrior Prep

This pose teaches us to do things in stages rather than rushing in without preparation.

- Begin in Three Legged Dog (see page 176) with your right leg lifted and as you exhale draw your right knee to your nose before stepping your right foot between your hands.

- Keep your left leg straight and hips low so your right thigh is parallel to the floor. Repeat on the other side.

Notes: If you can't get your foot all the way between your hands then get it as close as you can and then use a hand to lift the foot forwards.

Wheel

This is a strong backbend which will give you a sense of strength and freedom.

- Begin lying on your back with your knees bent and feet hip-distance apart. Reach your hands overhead and bend your arms to place your palms on the floor next to your neck with your fingers facing your shoulders.

- Push into your hands and feet at the same time and straighten your arms to lift yourself off the ground. Focus on lifting your pubic bone to the sky and pushing your chest between your arms.

Variations: If you have any back issues then avoid this pose and practise Baby Bridge (see page 132) instead.

Wide Legged Forward Bend

This pose gives you a beautiful stretch down your inner thighs and, because your head is below your heart, it will help shift your nervous system out of 'fight or flight' mode and into rest and digest mode.

- Begin in a wide stance and spread your arms out wide. Position your ankles underneath your wrists and bring your hands to your hips.

- As you inhale, lengthen your spine and as you exhale fold forwards, hinging from your hips, to bring your fingertips down underneath your shoulders in line with your toes.

- With each inhalation lengthen your spine and as you exhale fold deeper into the pose.

Wide Squat

This is a lovely way to stretch the inner thighs and release tension from the hips.

- Begin standing with your feet slightly wider than hip distance and turn your toes out slightly. Squat down to bring your bottom between your heels and your palms together in front of your heart with your elbows pushing your knees out.

Variations: If you are tight in your hips and find your heels lift off the floor then place a couple of yoga blocks or cushions under your heels to help you feel more stable.

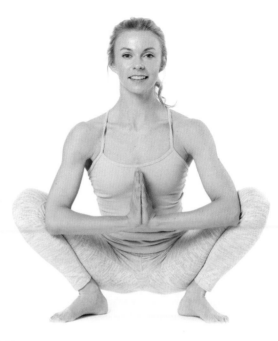

Wild Thing

Wild Thing helps you to explore the potential of your body and discover new strength and openness.

- Begin in Three Legged Dog (see page 176) with your right leg lifted. Open your hips and bend your right leg to bring your right heel towards your left buttock.

- Look under your left armpit and flip your Dog to bring your right foot to the floor as your lift your right arm and reach it overhead. Keep your hips lifted. Return to Down Dog (see page 144) and repeat on the other side.

Variations: If you have any shoulder issues avoid this pose. If you feel tight in your spine or shoulders, then stay in Three Legged Dog with your hips open and leg bent instead of flipping your Dog.

Windshield Wipers

This movement allows you to feel the freedom and space created in your hips from hip-opening poses such as Butterfly and Pigeon.

- Begin seated with hands resting behind you and your legs bent in front of you with your feet at least hip-distance apart.

- Let your knees fall from right to left a few times, aiming to get both knees touching the floor each time.

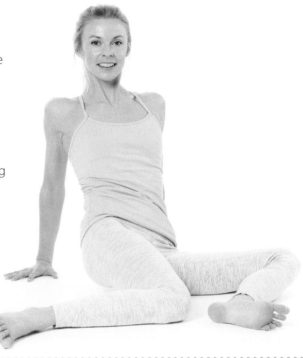

Winged Dragon

This is a beautiful pose to practise after Dragon Flying Low to increase the openness in your hips and help you feel more connected to your body.

- Begin in Dragon Flying Low (see page 145) with your right foot forwards and turn your toes out by 45 degrees so your foot is diagonal.

- Gently wing out from your right hip onto the little toe edge of your right foot. Hold it here passively, focusing on relaxing the muscles all around your hips, before standing the knee up and repeating with the left leg forward.

Acknowledgements

I've dedicated this book to you as a reader. To those of you who have ever felt like you don't belong. To those of you who battle with dark days and keep on going when life feels heavy. To those of you who have had many metaphorical bricks thrown at you but are now building something beautiful with them.

I've also dedicated this book to my Dad who lost his battle to cancer while I was writing it. Shortly before he died, I asked him what his best piece of advice was that I could carry with me for the rest of my life. He replied with two words, 'be kind'. So, Dad, I know I haven't always listened to your advice (I still haven't got around to learning about the off-side rule or the difference between Star Wars and Star Trek), but that piece of advice has become my mantra and this book is one way I hope to spread kindness around the world.

I would also like to acknowledge a few more people who have supported me on my journey and who, without their support, this book would not exist.

Firstly, my Mum, who has not only read several drafts of this book and corrected my apostrophe use more times than anyone should have to, but who never lost faith in me, even in my darkest moments.

Secondly, my twin sister, Rachel, who inspires me in more ways than she will ever know.

And thirdly my nephew, Finnley, who, as well as teaching me a heck of a lot about Lego, has taught me how to love unconditionally.

I also owe a big thank you to my best friend Lucy Waddell, who I met in the sand pit in our school playground when we were four years old and who never fails to be enthusiastic about my ideas, no matter how crazy or impossible they seem. And to my other school friends including Alice Hollingum, Neena Shea and Sarah Cadwallader, who stuck by me through my struggles.

I'd also like to acknowledge all the yoga teachers who I have learnt from over the years. I still can't get my foot behind my head, but I can promise to do my best to pass on everything I have learnt from my time on the mat to inspire more peace, compassion and connection.

I'd like to thank my weightlifting coaches, Mike Pearman, John Walton, Andy McKenzie and Adam Willis, who have not only taught me how to be strong on the lifting platform, but how to use that strength in life too.

And to Dr. Deepika Rodrigo and everyone at The Ayurvedic Institute UK who helped me to realise that I don't need to be ashamed of my journey any more.

I also owe a huge gratitude to everyone at Bloomsbury Publishing, especially my editors Charlotte Croft and Sarah Connelly who took a risk on publishing a book from a slightly hippy, handstand-loving yogi with a dream to fill the world with a little more love. And also to Glen Burrows, who took all the photography for this book, put up with my awkwardness in front of the camera and made me feel beautiful.

And to those of you, of which there are too many to mention, who were there when the walls were crumbling, who helped me see the beauty in my scars and who inspired me to eat the damn doughnuts without worrying about the size of my thighs. To those who fed my fire, who made my heart flutter, who joined me on my crazy adventures and who helped me discover what it means to be truly alive.

Helpful Contacts

To contact me, watch a video of the Thrive Sequence, listen to audio versions of the meditations, or continue your journey towards thriving see www.NicolaJaneHobbs.com.

You can also get in touch on social media:

Instagram: @NicolaJaneHobbs
Twitter: @NicolaJaneHobbs

Facebook page: Nicola Jane Hobbs

Use the hashtag #ThriveThroughYoga to share your journey.

If you need further support, the charities below can offer you information and guidance.

UK

Mind
Provide advice and support to empower anyone experiencing a mental health problem.
www.mind.org.uk

Rethink Mental Illness
Provide expert, accredited advice and information to everyone affected by mental health problems.
www.rethink.org

Anxiety UK
Promotes the relief and rehabilitation of those suffering from stress and anxiety disorders.
www.anxietyuk.org.uk

Beat
The UK's leading eating disorder charity.
www.b-eat.co.uk

OCD Action
Raises awareness and provides support and information to those with OCD.
http://www.ocdaction.org.uk

Action on Addiction
Help both those living with addiction, and those living with people who suffer problems of addiction.
www.actiononaddiction.org.uk

US

National Alliance on Mental Illness
America's largest grassroots mental health organisation dedicated to building better lives for the millions of Americans affected by mental illness.
www.nami.org

Anxiety and Depression Association of America
Provides resources and information on depression and anxiety disorders.
www.adaa.org

National Eating Disorder Association
The leading non-profit organization in the US supporting individuals and families affected by eating disorders.
www.nationaleatingdisorders.org

International OCD Foundation
Supports those affected by OCD and related disorders to live full and productive lives.
www.iocdf.org

National Council on Alcoholism and Drug Dependence
Provide support to those who need assistance confronting the disease of alcoholism and drug dependence.
www.ncadd.org

Research References

Part 1

Anderson, N. B., Nordal, K. C., Breckler, S. J., Ballard, D., Bufka, L., Bossolo, L., and Vella, A. (2010). 'Stress in America findings', in *American Psychological Association*, 9.

Coid, J., Yang, M., Ullrich, S., Roberts, A., & Hare, R. D. (2009). 'Prevalence and correlates of psychopathic traits in the household population of Great Britain', in *International Journal of Law and Psychiatry*, 32(2), 65–73.

Deshpande, P. B., Madappa, P. K., & Korotkov, K. (2014). 'Can the Excellence of the Internal Be Measured? A Preliminary Study', in Scientific GOD Journal, 5(5).

Dienstmann, G. (n.d.). 'Scientific Benefits of Meditation – 76 Things You Might Be Missing Out On'. Retrieved from liveanddare.com

'Dieting In 2014? You're Not Alone – 29 Million Brits Have Tried To Lose Weight In The Last Year' (2014). Retrieved from www.mintel.com

Dreisbach, S. (2011). 'Shocking Body-Image News: 97% of Women Will Be Cruel to Their Bodies Today'. Retrieved from www.glamour.com

Hefferon, K., Grealy, M., & Mutrie, N. (2008). 'The perceived influence of an exercise class intervention on the process and outcomes of post-traumatic growth', in *Mental Health and Physical Activity*, 1(1), 32–39. doi.org/10.1016/j.mhpa.2008.06.003.

Hoge, E. A., Chen, M. M., Orr, E., Metcalf, C. A., Fischer, L. E., Pollack, M. H., & Simon, N. M. (2013). 'Loving-Kindness Meditation practice associated with longer telomeres in women', in *Brain, Behavior, and Immunity*, 32, 159–63.

'How Common Is OCD?' (n.d.). Retrieved from www.ocduk.org

Kiecolt-Glaser, J. K., Bennett, J. M., Andridge, R., Peng, J., Shapiro, C. L., Malarkey, W. B., & Glaser, R. (2014). 'Yoga's impact on inflammation, mood, and fatigue in breast cancer survivors: a randomized controlled trial', in *Journal of Clinical Oncology*, 32(10).

McManus, S., Meltzer, H., Brugha, T. S., Bebbington, P. E., & Jenkins, R. (2009). *Adult Psychiatric Morbidity In England, 2007: Results Of A Household Survey*. Retrieved from www.sp.ukdataservice.ac.uk

Moore, P. (2015). 'Americans Are Tired Most Of The Week'. Retrieved from www.statista.com

Perälä, J., Suvisaari, J., Saarni, S. I., Kuoppasalmi, K., Isometsä, E., Pirkola, S., & Härkänen, T. (2007). 'Lifetime prevalence of psychotic and bipolar 1 disorders in a general population', in *JAMA Psychiatry*, 64(1), 19–28.

Ranscombe, S. (2015). 'British Women and the "Cult of Never Good Enough"'. Retrieved from www.telegraph.co.uk

Rosch, P. J. (2009). 'Bioelectromagnetic and subtle energy medicine', in *Annals of the New York Academy of Sciences*, 1172(1), 297–311.

Spinazzola, J., Rhodes, A. M., Emerson, D., Earle, E., & Monroe, K. (2011). 'Application of yoga in residential treatment of traumatized youth', in *Journal of the American Psychiatric Nurses Association*, 17(6), 431–44. doi.org/10.1177/1078390311418359.

Spurio, M. G. (2016). 'The new functional identity: a body that thinks, a mind that feels – Frontiers and unexplored territories of the "Body and Mind Zone"', in *Psychiatria Danubina*, 28(Suppl-1), 111.

Stambor, Z. (2006) 'Stressed Out Nation'. In *American Psychological Association*. Retrieved from www.apa.org

Tedeschi, R. G., & Calhoun, L. G. (1996). 'The Posttraumatic Growth Inventory: Measuring the positive legacy of trauma', in Journal of Traumatic Stress, 9(3), 455–71.

'Why Do Most Women Hate Their Bodies?' (2001). Retrieved from www.dailymail.co.uk

Wood, J. V., Perunovic, W. E., & Lee, J. W. (2009). 'Positive self-statements: Power for some, peril for others', in Psychological Science, 20(7), 860–66.

Part 3

Amin, A. (n. d). 'The 31 Benefits of Gratitude You Didn't Know About: How Gratitude Can Change Your Life.' Retrieved from happierhuman.com

Beck, M. (2012). 'Anxiety Can Bring Out the Best.' Retrieved from www.wsj.com

'Body Image Statistics' (n. d.). Retrieved from www.lookpositive.co.uk

Brooks, A. W. (2014). 'Get excited: Reappraising pre-performance anxiety as excitement', in *Journal of Experimental Psychology: General*, 143(3), 1144.

Brown, B. (2010). 'The Power of Vulnerability.' Retrieved from www.ted.com

Chevalier, G., Sinatra, S. T., Oschman, J. L., Sokal, K., & Sokal, P. (2012). 'Earthing: health implications of reconnecting the human body to the earth's surface electrons', in *Journal of Environmental and Public Health*, doi 10.1155/2012/291541.

Desan, P. (2010). 'Mihaly Csikszentmihalyi.' Retrieved from www.pursuit-of-happiness.org

Donnelly L. (2013). 'Almost half of Britons consider themselves "stressed".' Retrieved from www.telegraph.co.uk

Kellerman, J., Lewis, J., & Laird, J. D. (1989). 'Looking and loving: The effects of mutual gaze on feelings of romantic love', in *Journal of Research in Personality*, 23(2), 145–61.

Kuppusamy, M., Kamaldeen, D., Pitani, R., & Amaldas, J. (2016). 'Immediate Effects of Bhramari Pranayama on Resting Cardiovascular Parameters in Healthy Adolescents,' in *Journal of Clinical and Diagnostic Research*: JCDR, 10.5.

Meichenbaum, D. (2006). 'Resilience and posttraumatic growth: A constructive narrative perspective', in *Handbook of Posttraumatic Growth: Research and Practice*, 355–68.

Melnick, M. (2013). '20 Scientifically Backed Ways to De-Stress Right Now.' Retrieved from www.huffingtonpost.com

Morin, A. (2014). '7 Scientifically Proven Benefits Of Gratitude That Will Motivate You To Give Thanks Year-Round.' Retrieved from www.forbes.com

Neff, K. (n.d.). 'Exercise 3: Exploring Self-Compassion Through Writing.' Retrieved from self-compassion.org/exercise-3-exploring-self-compassion-writing/

'PSYCHO-ONCOLOGY: Discover How Prolonged Chronic Stress Causes Cancer and How to Heal Within.' (2012). Retrieved from www.alternative-cancer-care.com

Raidl, M. H., & Lubart, T. I. (2001). 'An empirical study of intuition and creativity', in *Imagination, Cognition and Personality*, 20(3), 217–30.

Seligman, P. & Peterson, M. (n. d.) 'The VIA Character Strengths Survey.' Retrieved from www.viacharacter.org

Seppala, E. (2014). '18 Science-Based Reasons to Try Loving-Kindness Meditation Today!' Retrieved from www.emmaseppala.com

Turner, K. (2014). 'The Science Behind Intuition.' Retrieved from www.psychologytoday.com

'What Can Mindfulness Do For You?' (n.d.) Retrieved from franticworld.com

Index

Page numbers in *italics* are poses; in **bold** are sequences.